TESTOSTERONE
SWITCH

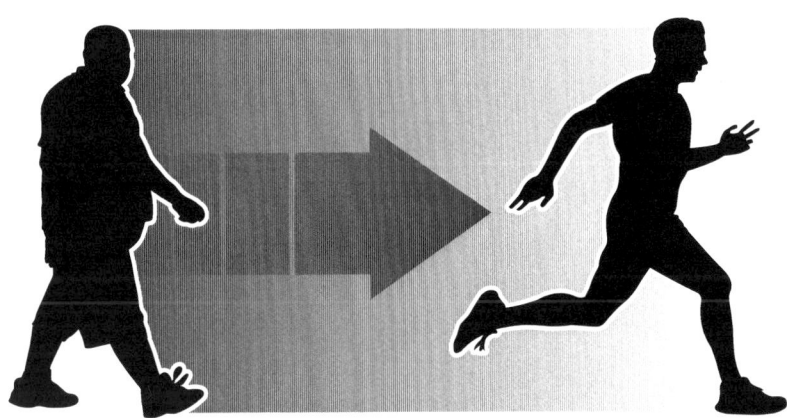

3 VITAL STEPS TO IMPROVE · LEAN MUSCLE MASS
PHYSICAL STAMINA · ENDURANCE · VITALITY · MOTIVATION
MENTAL PERFORMANCE · SPEED OF REACTION
SEXUAL FUNCTIONS · LIBIDO AND CAPABILITY

DR. KYL SMITH

The Testosterone Switch™

3 Steps To Naturally Increase Testosterone and Improve:

Lean Muscle Mass – Physical Stamina – Endurance
Vitality Motivation – Mental Performance – Speed of Reaction
Sexual Functions – Libido and Capability

Book and cover design by Ronald LaBelle, www.ronaldlabelle.com
Photograph of Dr. Smith by Shannon Drawe, www.sdphotography.com
Printed in the USA
Published by: Brighter Mind Media Group, Ltd. 4251 FM 2181 #230-515
Corinth, Texas 76210

www.TestosteroneSwitch.com

Dedication

To Kathy, my wife, best friend, and soul mate:

Thank you for your enduring faith in me. You provide the platform and environment that allow me to do the things I love to do. For the unwavering comfort and grounding presence you bring to my life I am truly grateful.

TABLE OF CONTENTS

Intro.

INTRODUCTION

400% INCREASE IN TESTOSTERONE!

"Since combining the testosterone boosting diet, daily exercise, and the nutritional supplements I'm about to share with you, my total testosterone quadrupled (that's right – increased four-fold over the first baseline blood level) while I gained lean muscle and lost 25 pounds of fat!" - Dr. Kyl Smith

In over 7,000 blood tests, one source reported "an epidemic of testosterone deficits" where "more than 80% of men tested had less than optimal testosterone blood levels."[1] ABC News, quoting *The Journal of Clinical Endocrinology & Metabolism* stated, "1 in 4 Men Over 30 Has Low Testosterone."[2,3] Conservatively, this translates to more than sixteen million men suffering with less than optimal testosterone in the United States today.[4] Nutritionally oriented physicians and nutritionists who are evaluating hormones in aging men often find otherwise healthy men in their 40's and 50's with *less than half the testosterone of a healthy 30-year old*.

So let me point out the obvious: If your testosterone is less than half of what it was when you were 30, then you probably feel like you're "less than half the man you use to be." Now keep in mind, I'm saying this because I can 100% relate! The 3-step plan you are about to learn was born out of my own sheer pain and necessity. That is, at just 45 years old, my testosterone was extraordinarily low at 195 ng/dL. If you are not yet familiar with "normal" testosterone values, let's begin by introducing you to the fact that "healthy 30 year olds often have total testosterone levels of approximately 700 ng/dL." *This means I was at about 27% of the healthy testosterone level of a 30 year old man – and let me tell you – I felt like it!*

As you can probably imagine, with a 20+ year background in nutritional research and a passion for exercise physiology I simply had to ask the question:

"Is there any science-based natural way to increase my own testosterone levels?"

Keep in mind, this was in fact a desperate search, as I really didn't like the idea of utilizing any outside source of testosterone that could potentially cause harm. Being mindful of the many listed side effects of common commercialized therapies my thought was: "I want to give it my best shot (no pun intended) to naturally increase my natural testosterone levels, and if that doesn't work, then I'll look closely at the 'other' options."

Well, the answer to that core question literally changed my life. It took me on a journey of discovery where I found an abundance of scientific references to support and prove that certain foods, targeted nutrition, and a very specific form of exercise would boost testosterone levels in young and older men. Even more, when you combine the three factors above (diet, nutrition, and exercise) there are complementary – even synergistic effects.

In the process I also discovered why testosterone production shuts down in men with low testosterone. Better yet – I learned how to "fix" it.

Since this discovery, I've traveled across the country and taught nutritionally oriented doctors how to implement the same 3-step protocol with their male patients to boost and improve testosterone in their practices. Of course today, I'm sharing this same science-based 3-step protocol or plan with you!

So let me begin with the most important statement I can make. If you are reading this text right now, you likely have "low" testosterone, and you are looking for a natural way to boost your own testosterone levels just like I was. Well, I want to reassure you and confirm you are in the right place. Even better, I want to share with you – *if you do have low testosterone –* ***absolutely nothing feels as good as boosting or increasing your testosterone levels!***

I've come to believe testosterone is practically like "oxygen" for a man. It is so fundamentally important for everything it is to be a man, that increasing or restoring low-sagging testosterone levels feels like it improves every aspect of your life – the way you think, feel, and move. In a myriad of ways your brain and body feel literally refreshed and respond positively to restoring and improving healthy testosterone levels. You have a lot to look forward to!

On the flip-side, "low" testosterone is a bane on mankind. "Why" is simple – ***low testosterone is a serious quality of life*** *issue for men*. When a man's testosterone levels are low, they experience **declines** in just about every category that defines true quality of life: energy, stamina, libido, muscle mass and strength, coupled with an **increase** in the daily experience of fatigue, tiredness, lethargy, lack of motivation and yes – weight gain.

Even worse, men with hormonal imbalances commonly suffer with an increased experience of prostate problems leading to frequent urges to urinate, lost sleep because of having to get up to urinate in the middle of the night, and difficult urination with dribbling, in other words – "benign prostatic hypertrophy (BPH)."

As men reach their 40s, most will start noticing subtle physical and emotional changes – soft spongy abdominal fat takes the place of hard muscle – and it seems regular physical exercise doesn't come close to producing the results it used to.

The Bane of Low T:

A man suffering with low testosterone typically experiences mild to moderate fatigue, lethargy, tiredness, or sapped motivation that just won't go away. Men contribute largely to the success of the "energy drink market" as they continually seek some form of artificial energy boost like caffeine throughout the day to attempt to feel "normal."

The problem is caffeine and energy drinks only serve to mask the fact that there's a lack of healthy anabolism, constructive metabolism, and healthy energy that permeates every aspect of the man's being. Other symptoms that men with low testosterone commonly suffer with are weight gain – especially abdominal fat, sagging physical stamina, loss of muscle tone, mild depression or mood swings, In other words they just don't feel like they did when they were motivated, energetic and young.

The good news is naturally enhancing this core hormone quickly and positively revitalizes every aspect of what it is to be a man – benefiting protein synthesis, enhancing skeletal muscle mass, bone density, and revitalizing mood, motivation, physical stamina, as well as improving cognitive functions like memory, mental performance, and speed of reaction.

Of course, healthy testosterone also improves sexual functions such as libido and capability as well as strengthens and sustains erections. The key here to put in more subjective terms – *restoring testosterone makes you feel like you did when you were younger, more energetic, and vibrant.*

In the pages that follow, you'll see the publicly available peer-reviewed science regarding healthy testosterone. Not only will you learn exactly what to do to naturally enhance testosterone, but I hope you are awed and inspired by the fact that there is so much that science says can be done utilizing diet, exercise, and nutrition to powerfully boost and restore testosterone levels in healthy men.

The Testosterone Switch 3-Step Plan Is Grounded In Science:

To stay true to the science, the technical expressions and quotes from scientific papers are often left intact. While this results in the book reading academically, I chose to go this route because it serves to best highlight the powerful statements made by researchers and scientists about this subject today.

This is important because the subject of "naturally boosting testosterone" is littered with questionable and dubious products. As a result, many men and health professionals are skeptical – and rightly so. To attempt to put the skeptics at ease, this book and the 3-step protocol within are grounded in science available at www.PubMed.gov (aka. The US National Library of Medicine / National Institutes of Health).

IMPORTANT NOTE:

In the "summary section" of this book you'll find a detailed, yet condensed and targeted plan including simple action steps to help you implement the Testosterone Switch 3-step plan. If you feel like "skipping to the summary," then please, feel free to do so! You can refer back to the wealth of science and scientific quotes in these pages at any time you wish for an explanation to exactly "how" and "why" the 3-step plan works. See page 91.

1

CHAPTER 1

"Low" versus "Healthy" Testosterone

To Begin, Here Are Some Science Based "Low Normal" Testosterone Facts:

- "Low normal" total testosterone concentrations are associated with reductions in energy, motivation, initiative, self-confidence, concentration and memory, sleep quality, muscle bulk and strength, diminished physical or work performance, feeling sad or blue, depressed mood, mild anemia, and increased body fat and body mass index.[5,6]

- Male sexual performance and function are dependent upon testosterone adequacy.[5-12]

- The strength, duration and quality of erections as well as the frequency of successful intercourse are proportional to serum testosterone concentration,[7-11] and successful erectile function is facilitated by testosterone.[12-20]

- Low normal serum testosterone concentrations increase the risk for premature death from any cause.[21-29]

- Low normal serum testosterone concentrations increase the risk for death from any cancer.[21]

- Low normal serum testosterone concentrations increase the risk for death from cardiovascular disease.[21,23,25,28,29]

- Low normal serum testosterone concentrations increase the combined risk for suffering a first stroke or first transient ischemic attack.[30]

- Low normal serum testosterone concentrations are associated with reduced male sexual desire, function, performance and potency.[5-11]

- Low normal serum testosterone concentrations increase the risk for memory loss.[31]

- Low normal serum testosterone concentrations increase the risk for developing clinical depression.[32]

- Low normal serum testosterone concentrations increase the risk for an increased level of systemic inflammation.[33-37]

Defining "Healthy" Testosterone:

What is a "healthy" or "normal" testosterone level in an otherwise healthy man? Well, the healthy ranges of normal serum testosterone concentrations remain controversial, especially when considering the incredibly positive impact of testosterone's influences on physiology over time.

In addition, there is a lack of consensus or agreement concerning the potential usefulness of calculating the serum concentrations of free testosterone (unbound testosterone) or biologically active testosterone (unbound testosterone plus testosterone bound to albumin).[38]

For this reason, The Testosterone Switch focuses exclusively on <u>total testosterone</u> values and reviews specifically the _health deficits_ of low and "low normal" testosterone, <u>compared to the many _health benefits_ associated with higher reference range, normal, _healthy testosterone_.</u>

While trying to arrive at a science-based definition for healthy testosterone it's worth repeating that _relatively mild testosterone inadequacy_ is associated with increased incidence of reductions in energy, motivation, initiative, self-confidence, concentration and memory, sleep quality, muscle bulk and strength; diminished physical or work performance; feeling sad or blue; depressed mood or dysthymia; mild anemia; and increased body fat and body mass index.[5,6]

This is important to revisit because there are multiple peer-reviewed papers that state <u>"testosterone deficiencies" and "desirable testosterone" in men is actually much higher than what is currently being considered as "normal" in doctor's practices across the country.</u>

In other words: The number of otherwise healthy men who suffer with "less than desirable testosterone levels" is shocking – and may be the #1 unmet need in aging men across the United States today! This means the number of men affected is likely twice the statistic quoted in the introduction of this book – potentially representing more than 30 million men!

Investigators examining the Framingham Heart Study Generation 3 (non-obese men aged 19 to 40 years with no history of any cancer, myocardial infarction, stroke, congestive heart failure, coronary surgery, peripheral angioplasty, diabetes, hypertension, hypercholesterolemia or smoking) characterized men with mid-morning serum total testosterone concentrations in the lowest 2.5th percentile for this cohort (less than 348 ng/dl) as "testosterone deficient," and stated that "low normal testosterone" is defined as total testosterone levels between 348 ng/dL and 406 ng/dL.[39]

In 2010 the Endocrine Society concluded that "low normal testosterone" is indicated by a mid-morning serum total testosterone concentration between 300 ng/dL and 400 ng/dL.[5] The 2010 Princeton Consensus Conference III associated "low normal testosterone" with mid-morning serum total testosterone concentrations between 230 ng/dL and 350 ng/dL.[40] The participants at this Consensus Conference also concluded that "desirable" serum total testosterone concentrations fall between 350 ng/d and 600 ng/dL.

Finally, in a cross-sectional study of Swedish men aged 69 to 80 years, the risk for premature death from any cause[26] and the risk for suffering a major cardiovascular event[27] were inversely correlated with the total serum testosterone concentration (i.e. the higher the testosterone levels, the lower the risk). Specifically with regards to cardiovascular events, men in the highest quartile of testosterone (at or higher than 550 ng/dL) had a lower risk of cardiovascular events compared with men with lower testosterone.[27]

More importantly, details from this study show that it did not matter if the men's total testosterone was very low (below 340 ng/dL) or moderately low (up to 549 ng/dL)…all men below 549 ng/dL had a similar increased risk for suffering a cardiovascular event. ***Only when total testosterone exceeded 550 ng/dL did cardiovascular risk drop…***

Now this is alarming as cardiovascular disease is the undisputed #1 killer of men in the United States and even more – this study was published in the *Journal of the American College of Cardiology!* These researchers documented a <u>*30% reduction in cardiovascular events*</u> as well as a <u>*decrease in cerebrovascular disease incidence*</u> – <u>where men with the highest total testosterone had a 24% reduced risk of transient ischemic attack or full-blown stroke.</u>[27]

Clearly based on this last quoted study, and the "desirable" serum total testosterone concentrations of the 2010 Princeton Consensus Conference III as stated above, potentially the only target for "healthy testosterone" is to maintain total testosterone <u>at or above 550 ng/dL</u>.

Now – allow me to point out something totally ridiculous and I believe, even harmful in men's healthcare today. The "healthy reference range" for total testosterone is 348 – 1197 ng/dL. This means it's just as "normal" to have a total testosterone level of 350 ng/dL as it is to have a total testosterone level of 1190 ng/dL. As a healthcare practitioner, and probably more important, as a 50 year old man who has suffered with low testosterone I can tell you for sure – *there's a world of difference in how you feel and perform (both mentally and physically) when your testosterone is "low normal" versus higher up the healthy "normal" reference range.*

So from my personal and professional experience with this subject, maintaining total testosterone levels at 750 ng/dL (about 2/3 of the "healthy reference range") can be achieved with a testosterone boosting diet, targeted supplementation, and a specific way to exercise; and is associated with significant enhancements and improvements in subjective perception of overall physical function, strength, vitality, energy, cognitive function, and mood.

LabCorp® Testosterone / Estradiol / DHEA-S Reference Intervals for Men	
Testosterone, Serum	348 – 1197 ng/dL
Free Testosterone	6.8 – 21.5 pg/mL
Estradiol	7.6 – 42.6 pg/mL
DHEA-S	44.3 – 331 ng/mL

Notes:
Always have your testosterone tested in the morning at or before 10:00 AM when it is typically at its highest daily level. Then, always retest at the same exact time.

Go to your healthcare provider and have all of the above hormone values evaluated, or go to www.DirectLabs.com for the best prices on laboratory testing.

In most states, DirectLabs.com does not require a doctor's requisition for the tests listed above. You simply pay with a credit card and follow the instructions to a LabCorp® destination near you.

2

CHAPTER 2

Estradiol versus Testosterone

As you'll see in the chart at the end of this short chapter, "healthy" estrogen (aka estradiol) levels are critically important for a man's health. The reality is, estradiol levels in a man need to be precisely balanced with testosterone in a very specific range. If estradiol levels rise, or testosterone levels fall, or both – this will wreak havoc on a man's health and even his life expectancy.

Aromatase, also called estrogen synthase, is an enzyme responsible for a key step in the biosynthesis of estradiol. In particular, aromatase is responsible for the aromatization of androgens (like testosterone) into estradiol. The aromatase enzyme can be found in adipose (fat) tissue and should be a huge consideration whenever a man has a beer-belly, excess belly-fat, love handles, or increased body-fat percentage.

Partly because whole-body aromatase activity is greater, and partly because older men typically have a higher percentage of body-fat, older men typically convert testosterone to estradiol *faster* than younger men.[41] Thus, in men serum estradiol concentration increases with increasing age[42] while the serum total testosterone concentration decreases with increasing age.[43-71] Consequently, an unbalanced ratio of estradiol to testosterone concentration increases with increasing age.[42,63]

Here's why this is a <u>big</u> problem for testosterone: In a man's testicles, Leydig cells generate testosterone via the process known as steroidogenesis. However, *the Leydig cells ability to generate testosterone is weakened in the presence of an increased ratio of estradiol to testosterone.*[72] This means an elevated ratio of serum total estradiol concentration to serum total testosterone concentration further exacerbates age-related decreases in testosterone synthesis and secretion.

Being that an elevated ratio of estradiol to serum total testosterone concentration has harmful consequences,[73-75] maintaining an appropriate balance between estradiol and testosterone is necessary in order to optimize overall health.[72-77] For this reason, it's critically important to measure estradiol when evaluating testosterone and work to maintain estradiol in balance.

It's also important to point out that *soy isoflavones* have estrogenic activity and directly inhibit the activity of several enzymes in the testosterone synthetic pathway. This means soy isoflavones have the potential to further reduce testosterone synthesis and secretion in men.[76] So, if your goal is to increase testosterone, completely eliminate soy isoflavones from your diet. Otherwise, you may begin to prefer spending your Friday nights with a cop of hot cocoa, Snuggies®, and a good date movie.

The Many Benefits of Healthy Estradiol Balance:

Estradiol is by far the most potent estrogen (10 times more potent than estrone, and 80 times more potent than estriol).

Men with low estradiol (the lowest 20% of the population [below 12.9 pg/mL]) are 317% more likely to die from any cause.

Men with high estradiol (the highest 20% of the population [above 37.4 pg/mL]) are 133% more likely to die from any cause.

The balanced estradiol quintile is 21 – 30 pg/mL. Men in this healthy range exhibit the greatest health benefits. An even better target for estradiol may be 21 – 25 pg/mL.

3

CHAPTER 3

Cortisol is The "Testosterone Switch"

Take a look at the picture painted by emerging research so far:

1. There are a significant number of men today suffering with testosterone levels below 550 ng/dL

2. With increasing age, there is typically an increase in estradiol and loss of balance between testosterone/estrogen.

Now add to that what you are about to see: An intricate dance unfolds between the stress-hormone cortisol, insulin, and testosterone, each interacting to affect glucose homeostasis, glucose uptake by muscle, an overactive dysfunctional "stress response," and most importantly – *significant interplay between each of these hormones synthesis and secretion.*

In fact, you are about to see that "<u>excess cortisol is the testosterone switch</u>" in a man's body – and controlling, mitigating, and limiting excess cortisol literally "flips a switch" allowing testosterone to be "turned on" and generated in healthy abundance again.

To begin, note that excess cortisol (known as *hyper*-cortisolemia) directly interferes with healthy insulin physiology. This is seen when healthy men exhibit fasting plasma glucose concentrations and degrees of insulin resistance that are *directly corre-*

lated with fasting plasma cortisol concentrations (i.e. when cortisol goes up, insulin goes up).[139,140]

In fact, fasting plasma glucose *and* insulin concentrations are directly correlated with fasting plasma cortisol concentrations,[78-81] and the degree of insulin sensitivity is inversely correlated with fasting plasma cortisol concentrations (i.e. higher cortisol levels raise insulin levels *and* lower insulin sensitivity).[78-81] So in essence, *hyper*cortisolemia is also a "diabetic switch" setting the stage for metabolic syndrome and diabetes in the future.

Why is this so important? You will soon see this subject ties directly into testosterone because a major factor for naturally generating "healthy testosterone" is maintaining a strict healthy balance of glucose and insulin. Said another way: Improving insulin sensitivity benefits testosterone as higher insulin sensitivity results in lower insulin levels, and ***low insulin is always associated with high testosterone***.

Cortisol Directly Inhibits Testosterone Synthesis

Acting through the classic glucocorticoid receptor, cortisol directly inhibits testosterone production in testicles by Leydig cells.[82-84] The cortisol-receptor complex suppresses testosterone synthesis via inhibition of the expression of the steroidogenic acute regulatory protein – *the very first step in testosterone synthesis*.[85] Even worse, *hyper*cortisolemia inhibits testosterone synthesis,[82-88] reduces the total testosterone concentration,[82-88] and accelerates the apoptosis (cell death) of Leydig cells.[88]

Oh yes – this should alarm you because it means:

A. Cortisol stops testosterone synthesis dead in its tracks at the very start of testosterone synthesis, and even worse,

B. Cortisol kills the cells in the testicles responsible for making testosterone in the future.

So "controlling *hyper*cortisolemia" is the key to generating healthy testosterone now *and* protecting your testicular Leydig cells so they can continue to do their job and make testosterone in the future.

Cortisol Stimulates the Activity of the Aromatase Complex

Even worse (if there can be such a thing), cortisol stimulates the activity of the aromatase complex in human male fibroblasts and adipocytes in fat deposits throughout the body.[89-92] Through this separate mechanism (completely different from inhibition of testosterone synthesis and secretion via Leydig cells as just described above), *hyper*cortisolemia increases the conversion of circulating testosterone into estradiol, increases the serum estradiol concentration, decreases the serum total testosterone concentration, and increases the ratio of the serum estradiol concentration to the serum total testosterone concentration in men.[82-84,86,87,89-92]

Acute Stress Increases Cortisol

What causes cortisol to spike!? In a word – *stress*.

Acute stress, whether psychological (mentally stressed at work, finances, home, family, etc.) or the result of a physical challenge (surgery, injury or intense exercise), induces a significant increase in cortisol secretion in healthy men.[93,94] For example, healthy men participating in a simulated job interview followed by a mental arithmetic test (real-world experiences designed to generate acute psychological stress), experienced a rapid significant increase in serum cortisol concentrations.[95]

Stress Decreases Testosterone

Stress-induced elevations in serum cortisol concentration are associated with rapid declines in testosterone production by Leydig cells in the testicles.[84] When male members of the ground crew of military aircraft were passengers on an acrobatic flight, they experienced acute anxiety that was accompanied by increased serum cortisol concentrations and decreased serum total testosterone concentrations.[96] Similarly, young men about to board an aircraft for their first skydiving attempt (a purely psychological stressor) experienced an acute increase in cortisol concentration and an acute decrease in total testosterone concentration.[97]

According to the American Psychological Association's Report: "*Stress In America*"

Americans Report that Stress Negatively Impacts their Physical and Psychological Health

Stress is a fact of life (agreed 79 percent of people), but according to survey responses, Americans routinely experience what they believe are higher than healthy levels of stress. One-third of people in the U.S. regularly report experiencing extreme levels of stress (32 percent), and nearly one in five (17 percent) report that they experienced their highest level of stress 15 or more days per month. Even more alarming, nearly half of Americans (48 percent) believe that their stress has increased over the past five years.

Three-quarters (77 percent) experienced physical symptoms during the last month as a result of stress. This includes fatigue (51 percent); headache (44 percent); upset stomach (34 percent); muscle tension (30 percent); change in appetite (23 percent); teeth grinding (17 percent); change in sex drive (15 percent); and feeling dizzy (13 percent), among others.

Nearly as many (73 percent) experienced psychological symptoms in the last month including irritability or anger (50 percent); feeling nervous (45 percent); lack of energy (45 percent); and feeling as though you could cry (36 percent).

Half (48 percent) of adults lay awake at night during the last month because of stress and on average they report losing 21 hours of sleep per month.

Ref: http://www.apa.org/news/press/releases/stress/

During exposure to spontaneously-occurring workplace psychological stress, 51-year-old men exhibited significantly decreased serum total testosterone concentrations.[98] Healthy men receiving painful electrical shocks also experienced an acute increase in cortisol concentration and an acute decrease in total testosterone concentration.[99]

Testosterone and Insulin Are Directly Related

Testosterone and insulin status are directly correlated.[73,100-108] Among adult men, the insulin secretion rate and fasting plasma insulin concentration were inversely proportional to serum testosterone concentrations (i.e. high insulin levels are associated with low testosterone, and low insulin levels are associated with high testosterone)[73,100] while whole-body insulin sensitivity was positively correlated with serum testosterone concentrations.[100,101] In other words, simple carbohydrates that evoke an insulin spike / increase will sabotage the production of healthy testosterone.

In the 10-year prospective observational 4th Tromso Study of middle age and elderly men, the men who later developed type 2 diabetes initially had lower mean serum total testosterone concentrations.[102] Among all of the men in this study, the risk for developing type 2 diabetes was inversely proportional to their initial serum total testosterone concentration (i.e. low testosterone significantly increased the risk for developing type 2 diabetes) and, compared to men with initial serum total testosterone concentrations less than 285 ng/dl, the risk for developing type 2 diabetes was reduced by about 60% among those men with initial serum total testosterone concentrations greater than 465 ng/dl.[102]

Testosterone and Insulin Facts:

- Testosterone and insulin status are directly correlated in non-exercising men.[173,100-108]

- The serum testosterone concentration and the fasting plasma insulin concentration are inversely proportional in non-exercising men.[173,100-108]

- Testosterone directly stimulates glucose uptake in muscle.[109]

- Increasing serum testosterone concentration increases insulin sensitivity in men.[173,100-108]

4

CHAPTER 4

Testosterone Switch Step #1:

Build Testosterone By Eating A Low Glycemic, Antioxidant Rich Diet

Since testosterone and insulin status are inversely correlated,[173,100-108] it's important to keep insulin low so testosterone will remain high. This makes diet imperative as some foods will spike insulin and glucose into the stratosphere wreaking havoc on healthy testosterone. Foods with a high Glycemic Index (GI) rating are those foods that are known to raise glucose and insulin concentration[110,111] and invariably drop testosterone like a rock. So in essence, the internal environment for healthy testosterone manifests when a man limits or eliminates high GI foods.

So what is a "high GI food?" Any food that spikes / increases insulin and blood sugar is a high GI food. As you would expect, table sugar (sucrose) and anything that contains it will rank high on the GI scale. So do foods made with refined flour and processed grains (white bread, pasta, white rice) or high GI sweeteners (such as honey, corn syrup, maple syrup) that produce larger increases in plasma glucose and insulin concentrations.[112,113]

Conversely, whole foods, including most fruits and vegetables (with the exception of white potatoes), have a much milder impact on blood sugar and insulin. For example, low GI foods (such as chickpeas, lentils, barley, leafy greens like spinach, lettuce, and fibrous vegetables like broccoli, cauliflower, asparagus) produce much smaller increases in plasma glucose and insulin concentrations. [112,113]

Investigators performing a meta-analysis of the published results of 45 intervention studies concluded that insulin sensitivity is inversely correlated with the glycemic index of an individual's habitual diet and that fasting insulinemia is directly correlated with the glycemic index of the habitual diet (i.e. high GI foods decrease insulin sensitivity and increase insulin). [114]

Furthermore, reducing the glycemic index of an individual's diet for just 4 days,[115] 7 days,[116] or 12 weeks,[117] produces an increase in the individual's insulin sensitivity and a decrease in the fasting plasma insulin concentration. This means in just 4 to 7 days an individual can improve insulin sensitivity and decrease insulin levels and thus, generate the internal chemistry that encourages healthy increases in testosterone.

More Information on "Low-Glycemic" Foods:

I've found that many individuals ask for more explanation on "the definition of a low-glycemic food." The key to understanding how to select low-glycemic foods is to understand which forms of carbohydrates best deliver sustained energy *without spiking blood sugar*. Ultimately this revolves around the sugar glucose, which is found in all carbohydrate foods, but *all carbohydrates are not created equal.* Some carbohydrates (carbs) are far better at fueling the body and healthy testosterone than others.

Unfortunately, nutritional information made available to "Joe-consumer" doesn't make a distinction between the carbs found in plant foods like apples, spinach, berries, tomatoes, or asparagus and those found in sodas, candy, sugar, refined cereals, biscuits, cakes and most other snack foods. "Nutrition Facts" panels on food labels handle these carbohydrates as if they are the same. *They aren't.*

Plant foods are made up primarily of carbohydrates, but they are *slow-releasing carbohydrates,* also known as *complex* carbohydrates (complex carbs). And to fuel testosterone, your body much prefers the steady source of fuel that *complex carbohydrates* provide, although your taste buds may be more attracted to the simple sugars found in cookies and sodas.

The dietary foundation for optimal healthy testosterone involves two (2) major factors:

1. Slow-release carbohydrates

2. Good-quality proteins

Slow-Releasing vs. Fast-Releasing Carbohydrates

Again, *slow-releasing* carbohydrates are the "good" ones aka *complex* carbohydrates, because their structure is bound to other complexes: other carbohydrates, phytonutrients (nutrient complexes in plants), antioxidants, vitamins, minerals, and fibers. Your digestive system has to dismantle these complex molecules to access the glucose they contain, which is quite a bit of work.

The end result is that complex carbohydrates are broken down into glucose by enzymes and acids and released into the bloodstream *steadily* and *gradually.* Unprocessed plant foods like fresh or frozen berries, most fruits, nuts, virtually all vegetables and unprocessed seeds, nuts, and whole grains are all sources of slow-releasing complex carbohydrates.

Fast-releasing carbohydrates are also called *simple* carbohydrates. (or *simple* sugars). Their structure is mechanically and/or chemically broken down into a concentrated, simple state by food processing—a sort of industrial pre-digestion. These processed carbohydrates cheat nature by isolating the sweetness in the food and discarding the rest. You can't cheat nature without consequences - and the super-sweet, super-harmful effects of refined sugar and flour are NOT exceptions to this rule.

When we concentrate sugars and discard naturally occurring fiber and nutrients that would slow their digestion down, we end up with white sugar and flour, brown sugar, malt, syrup, white bread, and other foods made with white flour like pasta, biscuits, and cereals. All of these are <u>fast-releasing</u>, <u>simple</u> carbohydrates—foods that are quite unlike the complex carbo-hydrates.

Because of the refining and milling processes, little work is required for these essentially pre-digested carbohydrates to be broken down by the digestive system. This causes them to be released <u>very quickly</u> into the bloodstream. The key concept here is this: *consuming fast-releasing simple-carbohydrates (simple sugars) causes a rapid increase in blood sugar and insulin levels that wreaks havoc on healthy testosterone.*

The Glycemic Index: Eating For Healthy Testosterone

So . . . what do you do? How exactly do you identify the fast-releasing carbohydrates that will spike your blood sugar into the stratosphere and drop testosterone like a rock?

A gentleman by the name of Thomas Wolever, M.D., Ph.D., from the Department of Nutritional Sciences and the Division of Endocrinology and Metabolism at the University of Toronto, has developed a concept that allows us to easily see which foods are the worst culprits when it comes to raising blood sugar levels.

Dr. Wolever's research identified that some foods create greater insulin demands on the brain and body than others, and wreak more havoc on the body's mechanisms for blood sugar control. He classified these foods with a *Glycemic Index* (GI) rating, which ranks foods based on their potential to raise blood glucose and insulin concentrations.[118] A high-GI food *greatly increases blood sugar and insulin levels* after eating.

As you would expect, table sugar (sucrose) and anything that contains it will rank high on the GI scale. So do foods made with refined flour and processed grains. Conversely, whole foods, including fruits and vegetables, have a much milder and controlled impact on blood sugar and insulin.

For your reference to comparative glycemic index values of different foods, Table 1 provides a list of the corresponding glycemic index values of some of the most commonly eaten foods.[119] To support the production of abundant, healthy testosterone, begin to eliminate the worst blood sugar offenders on the list. As you examine the list, one glaring point may leap out at you: the fact that most grain products produce a serious blood sugar and insulin response. When I first show this chart to people in lectures, they often share that they had not expected grains to be such bad news.

A telling example is corn flakes. This product produces a glycemic response that's literally off the charts! Notice, too, that bananas produce a high index. So think of this: Corn flakes, a chopped banana, adding a teaspoon of table sugar (sucrose)—how many men start their day with this combination or something similar and unwittingly suffer for it?

High-GI Foods Drop Testosterone

High-glycemic foods are the *worst* testosterone offenders of all. Foods with a high glycemic index disrupt hormonal balance, and imbalance your insulin levels far more than foods with a low glycemic index. High-GI drinks such as fruit juices and soda pop, beer, wine, liquor all trigger an undesirable blood glucose and insulin response in the body as well.

It's worth repeating: The result of eating high-glycemic foods will be an excess of insulin and glucose in the bloodstream. These excesses result in <u>low testosterone</u> plus, reactive hypoglycemia, poor energy, mood swings, and irritability. After repeated insulin spikes, the body begins to fail to properly adapt. Insulin resistance begins, with a list of degenerative conditions and age-accelerating symptoms soon to follow.

The answer to this dilemma is *balance.* You can begin the process of eliminating these blood sugar-related symptoms and reversing the progression of the health conditions with which they are associated by consuming *more low-glycemic* and *less high-glycemic* foods. In addition, you can dramatically slow down the release of carbohydrates and lower the glycemic index of foods with what I like to call the Glycemic Index-Protein Connection.

Glycemic Indexes of Commonly Eaten Foods

The following list includes over 75 foods categorized into five groups for simplicity and ease of use.

No GI—Lowest GI			
Cucumber	Radish	Artichoke	Asparagus
Spinach	Broccoli	Cauliflower	Eggplant
Celery	Cabbage	Green Beans	Lettuce—All Varieties
Berries—Raspberries, Blueberries, Blackberries	Peppers—All Varieties	Squash—Zucchini	Snow Peas, Bok Choy

Protein drinks: whey protein, egg protein, colostrum, | Seeds and nuts: almonds, flax, pumpkin, sesame, sunflower, walnuts, pecans | Lean meats: grass-fed beef, buffalo, poultry (turkey/chicken), fish, eggs | Fermented milk products: yogurt, kefir

Low GI (Good to combine with protein and/or nuts)			
Grapefruit	All-bran cereal	Peaches	Plum
Pears	Apples	Carrots	Chana dal
Chick peas	Grapes	Green peas	Kidney beans
Nopal	Oranges	Peaches	Cherries
Pears	Pinto beans	Red lentils	Strawberries
Cherries			

Medium GI (Large servings result in a high GI; limit portions and combine with protein and/or nuts)	
Apple juice	Bananas
Buckwheat	Fettucine
Navy beans	Orange juice
Parboiled rice	Sourdough wheat bread

Medium-High GI (Large servings will easily result in a high GI; limit portions and always combine with protein and/or nuts)	
Apricots	New potatoes
Wild rice	Pineapple
Sweet potato	

High GI (Any normal serving will easily result in a high GI; significantly limit portion or eliminate these foods. Alternative solution: Must combine with protein and/ or nuts!)	
White rice	Couscous
Life cereal	Sucrose
White wheat flour bread	Whole wheat flour/bread
Cheerios	Shredded wheat
Cornflakes	Baked Russet potato

The Glycemic Index-Protein Connection AKA: "The Testosterone-Sparing Effect of Dietary Protein"

Protein—it's not just for your muscles! Science shows that you can further balance your blood sugar when you *eat protein with carbohydrates.* This has been shown to effectively slow the release of the carbohydrate in the foods you are eating. If you choose to eat foods with a higher glycemic index, *combine them with lower-glycemic food choices.*

Here are a few easy examples:

- Eat seeds or nuts with fruit. For example: eat an apple, banana, orange, cherries, pineapple, apricots or grapes *with* a serving of walnuts, almonds, pecans or pumpkin seeds or "nut butters" made from any of the above.

- For breakfast, combine eggs with a serving of fresh berries and a dash of yogurt. Have your eggs cooked the way you like them, accompanied by fresh or frozen blackberries, raspberries or blueberries, with a table-spoon or more of yogurt on the side.

- Another example for breakfast could be the combina-tion of eggs with a serving of millet, buckwheat, or any whole-grain in general, plus fresh berries. In this case, try eggs cooked the way you like them, combined with organic buckwheat and fresh or frozen blackberries, raspberries or blueberries.

- Fresh raw pineapple with a veggie omelet may be the planet's most superior breakfast!

- For lunch, combine wild Alaskan salmon, free-range chicken, or grass-fed beef with a carotenoid-rich sweet potato and asparagus, salad, or another vegetable. The fiber and nutrients in the other vegetables, combined with the protein in the meat, will balance out the body's glycemic response to the sweet potato.

You Can Still Have Dessert!

An occasional sweet treat isn't going to harm your testosterone, but repeated overindulgences can and will contribute to a host of health problems. When you decide to indulge in something sweet, utilize the glycemic index to avoid foods that will overtly spike your blood sugar, or be sure to combine these foods with nuts and/or proteins that will slow the sugars' release.

The Building Blocks of Protein

High school biology class taught us—or, at least, *should* have taught us—that proteins make up the majority of our bodily tissues. The word *protein* was derived over 150 years ago from the Greek word *protos* or *proteios,* which you can find translated as both "first" and "of prime importance." Science has demonstrated that proteins are essential for growth and tissue repair and to act as carriers of important components in the blood.

Protein is the second most abundant substance in our bodies after water.[120] It constitutes as much as three-fourths of the dry weight of most body cells, with the exception of the brain, where the majority by weight is composed of lipids or fat.[120] The body utilizes proteins as building blocks for bone, skin, connective tissue, blood, and muscle.[120,121] They are major constituents of hormones and other chemical messengers, and are metabolically active in the form of enzymes that run, create, accelerate, limit and otherwise control all biochemical function throughout the brain and body.[120,121]

During digestion, proteins are broken down into their constituent amino acids, the basic building blocks of protein and of all living cells.[120,121] Different proteins are built from the 24 amino acids, bound together in various configurations.

All protein sources are made up of various combinations of these 24 amino acids. As such, proteins vary from simple to complex, incomplete to complete depending on the number, variety, volume, and order of amino acids in their structural chains. Like carbohydrates, *some forms of protein are more beneficial than others, based on the quality and quantity of specific essential amino acid units that make up the protein.*

What is a High-Quality Protein?

This book covers an exhaustive amount of information and references to show you how to boost and maintain healthy testosterone, but make no mistake: for optimal testosterone, food is first. I say this because no testosterone-boosting formula can make up for poor food choices in the foundational categories of carbohydrates, proteins, and fats over the long run.

For the most part, especially for those who do not restrict the types and combinations of proteins in their diets, protein is a simple subject. Unlike sugar, it's hard to eat the *wrong* proteins. There's really no such thing as a "bad" protein.

What are the best protein sources? You certainly have a lot of options. Perhaps the fairest and most practical way of rating proteins is to look for all of the *essential amino acids,* as well as how well the body utilizes and absorbs the amino acids in a given food.

This is essentially what nutritional scientists call the Protein-Energy Ratio (PER) and Biological Value (BV) ratings of proteins, which measure how well the body absorbs and utilizes amino acids in a protein. Let's look at a very short and generalized list of how the main protein sources rate (from highest to lowest) by looking strictly at how well they are absorbed and utilized in the body: their Biological Value ratings.

Protein:
Biological Value Ratings (BV)

Here is a short and generalized list of how the main protein sources rate (from highest to lowest) by looking strictly at how well they are absorbed and utilized in the body: their Biological Value Ratings (BV).

Excellent BV

BV 110–150	Whey protein isolates (protein supplements made at low temperature, containing non-denatured lactalbumin extract from dairy proteins, are the best source)
BV 105	Whey protein concentrates
BV 100	Egg white protein

You'll notice that of all the natural whole foods, nutritionists consider egg white protein to be the most perfect dietary source of protein for humans. Because egg whites are the "gold standard" against which all the other protein sources are compared, egg whites are given a BV of 100, which was essentially "perfect" until whey protein came along.

Whey protein is uniquely beneficial. It has immune-enhancing proper- ties and enhances the production of brain-protective glutathione; supports total body metabolism by stimulating the process of skeletal muscle protein synthesis; and stabilizes blood sugar levels (which is great for insulin and hence, testosterone).A protein with a biological value (BV) of 150 has twice the BV of a protein with a BV of 75. Your body will absorb and utilize the higher BV protein twice as efficiently. Simply adding one or two servings of "Excellent BV" proteins to your diet every day will provide the high-quality amino acids needed. As an example: I like to blend frozen blueberries with high-quality whey protein and sip on this in the morning or consume directly after a workout.

High BV

BV 95	Goat dairy products
BV 90	Cow dairy products
BV 85	Fish

Good BV

BV 80	Beef
BV 79	Whey protein concentrates
BV 77	Egg whites (from whole eggs)
BV 74	Soy (other than soy protein isolate) ††

For the sake of clarity, note that products labeled as just "soy protein" or "soy protein concentrate," tofu, and other soy-based products do not typically have a high BV. Soy is also low in the amino acid methionine and contains isoflavones, which as I shared earlier, are best to avoid.

Low BV

BV 59	Rice
BV 54	Wheat
BV 49	Legumes (beans, lentils)

Which Fruits And Vegetables Have The Most Antioxidants?

Scientists at the USDA set out to answer this question.[84] They utilized scientific method known as the Oxygen Radical Absorbance Capacity (ORAC) to analyze more than [100] different kinds of fruits, vegetables and other foods and determine their total antioxidant capacity per serving. Of the foods tested, here are best of the best: the foods with the very highest antioxidant scores. Be sure to eat lots of them on a daily basis!

Top Ten Highest-Antioxidant Fruits	ORAC Value
Blueberry (wild, "low bush" are best)	9019 (cultivated); 13,427 (wild)
Cranberry	8983
Blackberry	7701
Raspberry	6058
Strawberry	5938
Red Delicious apple (with peel)	5900
Granny Smith apple	4844
Cherry	4873
Gala apple	3903

Eat More Antioxidant Rich Foods

At the end of the day, naturally increasing testosterone in aging men is really about restoring youthful homeostasis (improving the regulation of hormonal conditions, so as to stabilize health and functioning). According to scientists, the biological and physiologic processes associated with aging and homeostasis reflect the rate of whole-body free radical production (oxidative stress)[122-126] and an imbalance in the body's oxidant and antioxidant status is an important etiologic factor for human degenerative diseases of aging.[122-127]

Free radical production (a deficiency in antioxidant status or an excess of oxidative stress) ties right into healthy testosterone as seen in this quote: "We conclude that aging is accompanied by reduced expression of key enzymatic and non-enzymatic anti-oxidants in Leydig cells leading to excessive oxidative stress and enhanced oxidative damage (lipid peroxidation). It is postulated that such excessive oxidative insult may contribute to the observed age-related decline in testosterone secretion by testicular Leydig cells."[128]

In other words, healthy testosterone is tied directly to healthy antioxidant status of Leydig cells in the testes.[128] Thus, significantly increasing consumption of dietary antioxidants and nutritional supplements that deliver potent antioxidant protection from free radicals is another key to increasing healthy testosterone. (Be sure to see the many benefits of Astaxanthin and Pomegranate extract in Chapter 6, on page 76).

5

CHAPTER 5

Testosterone Switch Step #2: Exercise With Intensity To Powerfully Boost Testosterone

It's been said that if you could put all the benefits of exercise in a bottle, you'd be the richest man in the world and I believe no truer words have ever been spoken. In fact, exercise packs such potent benefits there's simply no pill or potion that can beat it.

You will see that the immediate effects of one bout of intense exercise positively influences – *even "resets"* – the endocrine physiology of cortisol, insulin, testosterone, glucose homeostasis, glucose uptake by muscle, the "stress response," and improves rates of hormone synthesis and secretion and many metabolic and physiological systems that benefit healthy testosterone.

If you are out of shape don't worry, as even a single bout of intense resistance exercise performed to exhaustion by healthy untrained men produces an increase in serum total testosterone concentration.[129] And the more you exercise, the more benefits accrue to you as the effects of exercise on serum testosterone concentrations increase with continued training.[130]

Even more, exercise directly stimulates testosterone production as seen when healthy resistance-trained young men complete heavy resistance exercise. The induced increase in serum total and free testosterone concentrations are shown to result from an increase in testosterone synthesis within the testes.[131]

Exercise Improves Insulin Sensitivity

Previously you read that testosterone and insulin status are directly correlated,[73,100-108] and by that we mean – it's important to keep insulin low for testosterone to remain high. It turns out, exercise is another way to improve insulin sensitivity and reduce insulin levels. In fact, a number of experiments have examined the effect of an acute exercise bout on insulin physiology.

In many of these experiments, a single bout of moderate to high-intensity exercise (cycling,[132-137] running[137,138]) to exhaustion or near-exhaustion produced an immediate short-term increase in whole-body insulin sensitivity in healthy untrained men. For example, when men exercised on a cycle ergometer for 30 minutes at a moderate intensity workload or a high intensity workload, post-exercise insulin sensitivity was significantly greater than pre-exercise insulin sensitivity.[132]

Conditioning regimens as short as 7 days are as effective in increasing insulin sensitivity as are regimens lasting several months.[139,140] However make a note: The exercise-induced increase in insulin sensitivity is negated or abolished in overweight and obese men who continue to consume high GI diets.[138,141] So diet and exercise work hand in hand to decrease insulin and set the stage for increases in healthy testosterone.

Exercise Increases Testosterone (and Cortisol)

A number of experiments have examined the simultaneous acute effects of an exercise bout on cortisol and testosterone physiology in men. In these experiments, a single session of moderate to high intensity exercise (weight lifting,[142,143,146-148,150,151] jump squats,[146] rowing,[149] swimming,[149] cycling[144,145]) to exhaustion or near-exhaustion produced immediate short-term increases in serum cortisol and total testosterone concentrations[142,143-149,151] and in serum cortisol and free testosterone concentrations[142,143,146,147,150] in healthy untrained[142-146,150,151] and exercise-trained men.[147-149]

Note that in the studies quoted above, *both* cortisol and testosterone increased as a result of moderate to high intensity exercise. Next you'll see according to peer-reviewed science – there *is* a way to acquire the benefits of testosterone while keeping excess cortisol in check! Methods to accomplish this are explained in Chapter 6: "The Testosterone Switch Step # 3" just a few pages away…

The Benefits of Exercise Go Way Beyond What You'd Expect

You've just seen that intense exercise improves insulin levels and insulin sensitivity, increases testosterone, improves glucose homeostasis and glucose uptake by muscle, and improves rates of hormone synthesis and secretion and many metabolic and physiological systems that benefit a healthy body. In addition, intense exercise benefits and stimulates brain function including stimulating the anterior pituitary gland that sits in the middle of the brain.

The significance here is, in response to *intense* exercise, the anterior pituitary gland produces the anabolic elixir of life – *growth hormone*, while regulating stress, and secreting several peptide hormones that act on target glands like the adrenal glands and testicles. To get to the many benefits of growth hormone, let's first explore how exercise stimulates the brain and thus, growth hormone secretion.

In animals, exercise significantly increases the density of blood vessels in the brain.[152,153,154-156] This facilitates neuron function and long-term neuron survival in the parts of the brain responsible for motor learning,[156] which of course improves motor coordination and balance. In humans, the results are even better. *High-intensity exercise*—hard exercise that occurs when you really push yourself, like a full-on 100 yard dash that gets your heart pounding, gasping for air, and your body pouring out sweat—*results in increased cerebral blood flow,*[157-160] thereby increasing cerebral nutrient and oxygen supply and producing global brain benefits.[161,162]

As exercise intensity increases, blood flow is increased to all regions of the brain.[156] The increase in cerebral blood flow is sustained throughout the duration of physical activity.[163]

The take-home message is: *intense* exercise is better for both your body and brain.

The Many Benefits of Exercise: From The Research Front

In the research, you'll see that some studies focus on the *acute* effects of exercise and others on the *chronic* effects. The former type of exercise evaluates the effects of a single bout, during, or closely following, the workout; and the latter type evaluates the effects of repeated exercise sessions over a period of time.

Acute physical exercise has been found to:

- Increase task learning ability,[164] and performance on tests of concentration.[165,166]

- Increase post-exercise mental performance,[167] verbal adaptability,[168] verbal diversity[168] and verbal originality.[168]

- Improve reaction time in athletes who had just completed an exhausting exercise bout.[169]

- Significantly stimulate logical memory[196] and improve creative thinking.[197]

Chronic exercise leading to physical fitness has been found to:

- Increase long-term cognitive performance, cognitive ability and mood in adults of all ages. For example: a small 10 percent improvement in cardiovascular fitness was associated with significantly improved mood and cognitive function,[170] while improvements in fitness of 15 percent or more are associated with significantly increased short-term memory and speed of recall. The 15 percent increase in fitness also significantly reduced reaction time (meaning, you think quicker and faster), suggesting that information processing speed had accelerated.[178]

- Reduce mental reaction time (again, thinking quicker and faster)[171,172] and significantly increase learning ability[179] and decision-making capacity.[179]

- Improve working memory, reasoning ability, motor performance and reaction speed (this translates to improved athletic performance).[173-175]

Exercise and Growth Hormone: The "Master Hormone"

By now you've heard commercials on radio and television purporting the benefits of growth hormone. It's potent, powerful, youth-enhancing, muscle-boosting, athletic performance enhancing, that's certain. It builds and preserves hard, strong muscle; helps to burn excess body fat; heals tissue damage throughout the body; maintains youthful skin and dense bones; and helps you feel energetic and happy. The good news: you don't have to buy anything or take any pill or potion to increase your growth hormone levels. You can make your own . . . with exercise.

Before we get more deeply into the *how* of making more growth hormone, let's have a look at the *why*.

The Many Benefits Of Growth Hormone

Growth Hormone (GH):

- Reshapes the body. GH significantly stimulates protein synthesis, effectively increasing lean muscle mass and metabolism, and speeding the rate at which the body heals.[222–229,236,237,239,240]

- Melts away fat. In every study of its effects on normal, aging people, supplemental GH reduced body fat and increased lean body mass. *GH may be the most effective fat-loss agent ever discovered.*[223–235]

- Improves brain function. GH boosts energy levels, improves sleep quality (this is critically important for testosterone synthesis), elevates mood, reduces stress (again important for testosterone), improves focus and concentration, and improves self-esteem and self-confidence.[241–246] In addition, GH can reverse declines in memory and cognitive performance.[247]

Aside from the strong evidence linking regular physical activity to neurogenesis (increases of brand-new healthy new-neurons in the brain), enhanced cognitive and memory functions, and increased growth hormone secretion, physical exercise is a potent stimulator of other brain-body enhancing factors like *neurotrophin* and *insulin-like growth factor 1* (IGF-1).

IGF-1 has anabolic effects meaning, it "builds up" lean skeletal muscle while it sends extraordinarily "healthy" signals to specific insulin receptors helping to regulate and improve insulin sensitivity (as you recall, this is critically important for healthy testosterone). IGF-1 is a primary mediator of the beneficial effects of GH, it increases neurogenesis and improves cognitive functions in old animals,[254] improves neuromotor function, learning ability and memory retention in brain-injured adult animals[255] and reduces cerebral neuronal loss after injury.[256]

With this said, allow me to point out that most studies show that in order to get all of these GH-related benefits, you have to *exercise*. Don't think that any product said to "stimulate GH production" will result in all (or any) of the benefits detailed in this chapter. We haven't reached a total understanding of the ways in which exercise, hormones, neurotransmitters, and neural changes interact, but we do know that the whole equation is very complex. It can't be reduced down to effects of a single hormone, and certainly not a single product.

Workout Intensity: The Key To Boosting GH and Testosterone With Exercise

Young adults, older adults and elderly adults exhibit increases in plasma GH concentrations during and immediately following exercise sessions. These elevations in GH production are *proportional to the duration and intensity of the exercise session.*[180–201] In other words, *the more intense the exercise session, the more GH is produced in response*.

In order for plasma GH concentrations to increase in response to an exercise session, a threshold level of exercise *intensity* must be exceeded such that the exercise is *challenging* to the individual's level of physical fitness.[181,202–204] This gives further credence to the benefit of a challenging exercise session over one that just gets you moving a little faster than your usual sedentary state. It also means that as you become physically fit, you'll need to continue to keep the exercise sessions physically challenging.

The best kind of exercise for raising plasma GH concentrations is *intermittent exercise at this high intensity threshold*. Intermittent bouts of high intensity work, alternating with periods of lower (but still moderate, to moderately high) intensity, raise plasma GH better than continuous exercise performed below, at, or even above this threshold.[207–215]

This is possibly the most important research finding to date regarding the ability to naturally release GH during exercise. *High-intensity, intermittent exercise is the most rewarding for your brain and body!*[207–215]

Note that as you become more fit, your plasma GH response to exercise is never blunted by adaptation. In fact, your ability to release GH as a result of high-intensity exercise becomes more and more efficient over time, rewarding you more and more with every exercise bout.

Regular and consistent exercise programs will result in significant and consistent elevations in nighttime GH secretion and 24-hour integrated plasma GH concentrations.[203,219,220] This means that the more you consistently exercise, the more your brain and body will experience the benefits of healthy GH floating around, healing and repairing your cells, glands, organs and tissues.

Trudging along on a treadmill for 30 to 40 minutes or more at a constant pace <u>will not optimally release GH</u>.[207–218] I can't tell you how many times my heart has gone out to overweight men and women as they trudge along on treadmills for long, drawn-out, painful exercise sessions. These people probably end up wondering why they are not losing the weight they wanted to. They may question whether exercise is even worth the effort. Now you won't fall into that trap!

Intermittent exercise to your personal peak threshold is the key to making the powerful metabolic and hormonal improvements that will quickly take you to your fitness goals. So if your goal is to increase testosterone and growth hormone, build and tone muscle, lose weight, and significantly improve your mental function, and to do all of this as fast as possible with as little investment in time as possible, then intermittent exercise to our personal peak threshold is the best way.

Here's how to do it…

"Burst" or Interval Exercise: Intermittent Exercise To Your Personal Peak

This section is dedicated to showing you how easy it is to exercise in a *burst* fashion—also known as *interval training*—for maximal growth hormone release. Keep in mind that *you don't have to exercise in this way to benefit from exercise. But if your goal is to boost GH and testosterone, then this is your recipe for success!*

Any improvement you make in your fitness level will improve mental and physical function. Burst exercise is simply a way to *optimize* the benefits of producing maximal GH and testosterone in a completely natural and health-optimizing way.

Step One: Purchase a heart rate monitor at any local store that sells fitness or athletic equipment. This should be easy; almost all sporting goods stores carry them. You don't need a lot of "bells and whistles" on the model you choose, and you don't have to spend a lot of money. My favorite brand is Polar®. Expect to spend $50–$75.

Step Two: Review all of the information that comes with your heart rate monitor. Your goal is to know the exact values for 70 percent, 80 percent, 85 percent, and 90 percent of your maximal heart rate for your age.

Step Three: Have your physician review your health and make absolutely sure they are in agreement with your utilizing your heart rate monitor to intermittently exercise up to 70 percent, 80 percent, 85 percent, or 90 percent of your maximal heart rate for your age. Based on your level of health, your physician will let you know whether you can safely exercise at up to 90 percent of your maximal heart rate for your age—a level that is not dangerous, as long as your physician says it is appropriate for you and your level of health.

Step Four: After obtaining your physician's approval and determining your upper heart rate limit, select a method of exercising: swimming, cycling, Versa Climber®, mini-trampoline, punching bag, elliptical machine, running on a soft surface, or whatever other activity appeals to you. Use your Heart Rate Monitor to become familiar with your heart rate and how you feel when exercising. Give yourself seven days or so (five to six exercise sessions) to improve your fitness level by exercising at about 70–75 percent of your maximal heart rate.

Step Five: You're ready for the burst! After your initial five or six exercise sessions, begin an exercise session by warming up to about 70 percent of your maximum heart rate. Warm up for about two minutes by sustaining the 70 percent value. After warming up, sprint/burst as fast as you comfortably can, up to about 80 percent of your maximum heart rate. When you each 80 percent, rest and recover by breathing deeply as you slow or stop the activity. After your heart rate drops to about 70 percent, repeat the process: sprint/burst up to about 80 percent of your maximal heart rate.

When you reach 80 percent, rest and recover by breathing deeply as you slow or stop the activity. Repeat for a total duration of 10–15 minutes. Cool down and stretch when you're done (stretching at the end of your session serves to improve flexibility and joint range of motion).

A Specific Example of a Burst Exercise Session

Mini-trampolines are probably in stock at your local sporting goods store. They generally cost around $50, and provide an awesome way to exercise at home in a low-impact fashion. If you have access to one of these mini-trampolines (at home or at the gym) burst exercise is a snap. After putting on and turning on the heart rate monitor:

1. Begin to gently run in place on the mini-tramp. Your heart rate will rise to about 70 percent of your maximal heart rate. Sustain a couple of minutes at 70 percent to warm up. Note: Be sure to wear running shoes that fit well.

2. After your warm-up, sprint/burst by running in place as fast as you can (in a controlled and balanced manner) until your heart rate reaches 80 percent of your maximal heart rate. When you reach 80 percent, rest and recover by breathing deeply as you slow or stop the activity. If you wish, you can step off the mini-tramp and stretch and breathe deeply.

3. After your heart rate drops to about 70 percent, sprint/

burst by again running in place on the mini-tramp as fast as you can (in a controlled and balanced manner) until your heart rate reaches 80 percent of your maximum heart rate. When you reach 80 percent, rest and recover by breathing deeply as you slow or stop the activity. Repeat! Your total exercise session (including warm-up) should be 15 to 20 minutes ...

What You Can Expect With Burst Exercise

Studies that review the benefits of this kind of intermittent exercise show that high intensity exercise at intermittent intervals is significantly more beneficial than aerobic exercise at a constant pace with regards to improving GH, Testosterone and overall metabolism. [181,202–204,207–218,221]

- 10 to 15 minutes of burst exercise may be as effective as 20 to 40 minutes of aerobic exercise in terms of improving heart health and producing a positive hormonal response.[209,211,213,221]

- You can actually get the benefits of exercise in about 10 to 15 minutes a day when you are exercising with intensity. So there's no more excuses about not having enough time to work out—*everyone* has 10 to 15 minutes a day to spare - especially for these benefits!

Why I Want You To Visit With Your Physician Before You Begin

I don't want to give the impression that burst exercise is in any way dangerous for your heart or your health. In fact, it's a heart-healthy way to exercise when you are already in shape, and fit individuals who engage in sprint-type activities often bring their heart rate into high intensity zones.[181,202–204,207–218]

With this said, however, this form of exercise is not going to be appropriate for every individual who reads this book.

As an example, if you haven't exercised in years, then it's not a good idea for you to just slam into an intense exercise regimen. No matter how "fit" you think you already are, have your physician review your current level of health and make sure the types of exercise and intensity level you choose are right for you.

If your physician doesn't immediately say that intermittently exercising at 80 percent, 85 percent, or 90 percent of your maximal heart rate for your age is a good idea for you, hire a personal trainer to provide specific guidance that's customized to your needs. Tell your physician and personal trainer that your goal is to eventually do burst or interval exercise, and they can guide you to that goal in a step-by-step fashion that's right for you and your level of health. Please don't cut any corners here. Visiting with your physician first is of the utmost importance.

Effects of Exercise in the Prevention and Treatment of Depression

Duke University Medical Center has contributed greatly to the body of evidence that shows an anti-depressant effect of exercise—and improvements in cognitive ability—of middle-aged and elderly men and women.

For example, researchers at Duke University found that riding a stationary bicycle, walking, or jogging just three times a week for 16 weeks resulted in significant improvements in standard measurements of depression. The results demonstrated that exercise is just as effective as medication in treating major depression in some people.[247]

To date, the evidence that shows exercise can improve mood and alleviate depression is quite impressive:

- Participation in moderate aerobic physical activity benefits the "general mental health" of non-depressed adolescents,[278] adults of all ages[170,177,279–297] and elderly individuals.[295–300]

- Positive responses to regular physical activity include feelings of increased calmness and pleasantness and decreased anger.[301–304]

- Regular, moderate aerobic exercise has been reported to significantly reduce the risk of developing depression.[174,305–307]

- A chronically low level of physical activity may *increase* the risk of depression.[305,308] In one study that compared adults who exercised regularly with those who did not, the odds ratio for depression demonstrated a significant risk for depression among the non-exercising segment of the population.[307]

- In another group of adult women aged 25 to 77 years, being physically inactive doubled the risk for developing depressive symptoms within eight years.[306]

- Regular, moderate intensity exercise appears to improve the ability of adults to cope with emotional stressors.[295,309-313] For example: participation in a physical training program increased the ability of nurses and nursing aides to adapt to working overnight.[314]

- Highly active, non-depressed individuals who later develop mild depression have a lower likelihood of progressing to severe depression.[315]

- Exercise also has been reported to prevent the depressive symptoms induced by several pharmacologic agents.[316-320]

- By contributing to weight control and management, exercise may reduce the depressed mood common among the obese.[321-322]

- An overwhelming number of studies show that adults with clinical depression have exhibited reductions in depressive symptoms following aerobic exercise or strength training, even without evidence of measurable improvement in cardiovascular or overall physical fitness [281,284,285,287,288,293,295,299,306,310,312,315]

- Symptoms of anxiety and panic disorder also improve with regular exercise. [288,293]

- Aerobic exercise has been reported to be as effective as antidepressant medications in reducing the severity of depression. [292-296]

To Exercise Is To Improve

The word *exercise* is derived from a Latin word that means *to maintain, to keep,* or *to ward off.* Basically, exercise means to practice, put into action, train, perform, use, and even improve.

Physical exercise and activity have always been a natural part of life, although these days we have to consciously include it, plan for it, and make it a part of our daily routines. As you have seen, the benefits of exercising are profound, to say the least!

A few final points for this subject:

- Be sure to purchase a heart rate monitor. This device is beneficial whether you decide to do high intensity exercise or not; it allows you to accurately see the work your heart and body are actually doing. I feel strongly that this is just as important for someone who may accidentally overwork, as it is for someone who may *under*work and fall short of the results they could and should achieve. Knowing how your body is reacting to the exercise you are doing is an easy key to long-term success.

- The absolute best time to exercise is in the afternoon or early evening. If this window of time doesn't work with your schedule, then exercising in the morning is also good. The absolute latest you should exercise is about three to four hours before you plan to fall asleep. Exercising in the morning, afternoon, or at least four hours before you fall asleep supports your circadian rhythms and helps induce deep, restful sleep.

- Please note that if you choose to do "burst or interval exercise," then 10–15 minutes a day of intense exercise is all you need five or six days per week to maximize GH, testosterone, and all of the benefits of exercise. As such, for these kinds of rewards, you may be able to work 10—15 minutes of intense exercise into your morning, afternoon, or early evening after all!

- Remember: Obtain your physician's approval before engaging in high-intensity exercise.

Stress Drops Testosterone, But Exercise Protects Your Body From Stress

The rise in blood cortisol levels that results from chronic stress is a BIG problem when it is unopposed by growth hormone (GH).[209–212] Since exercise results in increased levels of GH and intense exercise results in significantly elevated levels of GH and testosterone, exercise powerfully blunts the negative effects of stress. In fact, you could say that the more intense the daily stress, the more intense your daily exercise program should be to effectively counter it.

The key here is that the stress hormones are not designed to work in isolation. Think about it for a moment. The "fight or flight" response was designed to result in an immediate "burst" of physical activity. Whether you were engaged in a "fight," or a quick "flight" was your goal, either way, you were physically active—probably to your physical limit. You might have been running from a grizzly bear in the woods, chasing down what you hoped would be dinner with all your strength and might, or protecting your loved ones from some kind of danger.

Let's say you started your day stuck in traffic, worrying about the mortgage (*stress-hormone cortisol is released*). Then, stuck in a board meeting with your big-sugary-grande-gulp coffee, you realize for the first time that your company is going down the tubes and your boss is doing his best to blame you (*more cortisol released*). Now you're really worried about the mortgage (*a veritable cortisol flood*). And there you sit, unable to fight or flee—and either response would give your body and brain a protective jolt of GH and testosterone.

At the end of a colossally stressful day like this, if you make it a point to release GH through physical exercise, the GH will, in effect, boost IGF-1 (improving insulin sensitivity), boost testosterone, and serve to protect *your brain, neurons, and body from the effects of elevated cortisol.* [209-216] In essence, you will have completed the fight-or-flight hormonal cycle and told your cells that they can finally cool down and relax.

The type of exercise that you pick is key if your goal is hormonal recovery. It appears that long duration and lower intensity cardiovascular exercise may improve mood and decrease depression (this is good), but may not fully solve the cortisol problem because these forms of exercise are not likely to oppose cortisol with significant amounts of GH and testosterone. This likely explains why standard aerobic programs are not as effective for weight loss or optimal body composition when compared to types of exercise that produce a larger GH, IGF-1 and testosterone responses.[241–244, 247,323]

Engaging in intense, short-duration physical exercise that optimally produces GH and testosterone is a powerful key to eliminating the negative effects of stress and the resulting glucocorticoids like cortisol.

It's All Connected: Exercise, Sleep, Testosterone, Mood and Memory

The field of neuroscience has established that sleep is not only crucial to brain development, but is also necessary to help consolidate the effects of waking experience. It turns out that sleep assists the conversion of memory into a neurologically permanent, readily accessible form.

What's this got to do with testosterone? It turns out rapid-eye-movement (REM) sleep is required for the consolidation of long-term memory *and the optimal production of testosterone.*[327–331] The storage of long-term memory requires biochemical modifications and the stimulation of certain neural pathways, and REM sleep facilitates both.[332–334] REM sleep deprivation significantly impairs memory-dependent learning and mental performance and drops testosterone.[330,331]

What does science say about the effect of daily exercise on quality of sleep? *To date, every study that has evaluated the positive effects of exercise on sleep has shown consistent patterns of improved sleep in those who take up an exercise program.*

It appears that a higher intensity of exercise may be best for improving sleep. Exercising at least three hours before bedtime is better than late evening exercise. However, in every case, some measures of improved sleep were consistently found with the addition of an exercise program, no matter the intensity or duration, and no matter what time of day. Any improvement in level of physical fitness results in improved quality of sleep.

Researchers have concluded that:

- Exercise improves sleep quality, sleep pattern, REM sleep, and decreases wake after sleep onset in healthy young good sleepers.[345]

- Exercise improves sleep pattern, REM sleep, and metabolic profile in elderly people[344]

- Those with moderate sleep complaints can improve self-rated sleep quality by initiating a regular, moderate-intensity exercise program.[339]

- Older adults with moderate sleep complaints can improve self-rated sleep quality through a moderate-intensity exercise program. In fact, exercise appears to be effective as another non-pharmacological approach to sleep enhancement for sleep-disturbed elderly individuals.[340]

- Healthy adults aged 49 and up can benefit from initiating a regular moderate-intensity exercise program; they see reductions in stress-induced cardiovascular reactivity and improvements in their ratings of their own sleep quality.[341]

- A study of depressed individuals showed that weightlifting exercise significantly improved all subjective sleep quality and depression measures.[342]

Sleep Is Key

It's really this simple: If you're not getting a minimum of seven or even eight hours of sleep most nights, you're *not* maximizing REM sleep, thus your *not* maximizing testosterone and you are putting your future health at risk. Even mild sleep deficits—like six hours a night for several nights in a row—will result in *measurable decreases in the ability to learn new information*. And missing sleep doesn't just make you feel slow – it can cause *long-term damage* to brain cells. The main point here is *sleep is not a luxury*. It's an important part of normal brain and body function. So any employer who requests that you "catch that red-eye" or "burn the midnight oil" on a regular basis doesn't have your—or even their best interests in focus when it comes to short-term or long term performance. Be wise—make at least seven to eight hours of sleep every night a non-negotiable necessity.

Here are more reasons why: During sleep your brain shifts attention (so to speak) to cellular housecleaning – basically cleaning out waste products. If you don't regularly get enough sleep, this vital work will not get done. Moreover, poor sleep habits markedly decrease immune function, and there is simply no such thing as a good mental or physical performance if the immune system is weak. Lack of sleep is also linked to depression, irritability, and anxiety – but you already know that because you've experienced it. So how do you get sleep back on track?

Exercise exactly as described in this chapter of the book. Daily exercise is one of the most potent and powerful ways to *reset, support, and strengthen* normal circadian rhythms (the normal "sleep–wake cycle"). Make a 30-day commitment to "test this principle." I promise you'll be glad you did!

Dr. Kyl Smith

6

CHAPTER 6

Testosterone Switch Step #3: Nutritional Supplements Control Cortisol, Aromatase, and Oxidative Stress to Build Testosterone

Since combining a low-glycemic diet, daily intense exercise, and the nutritional supplements I'm about to share with you, my total testosterone quadrupled (that's right – increased four-fold over the first baseline serum level) while I gained lean skeletal muscle and lost 25 pounds of fat. Even better, for five years now, as long as I remain consistent with the three-step program, I've always sustained the high healthy testosterone level of 720 ng/dL or higher. This third step, daily supplementation with nutrients that help control aromatase, cortisol, and provide antioxidant benefits is critically important to the success of the protocol in my experience.

Science clearly shows that excess cortisol is the enemy of testosterone. If a man is psychologically stressed (stress at home, work, finances, family etc.) or physically stressed (as with physical work or exercise) excess cortisol derails his ability to generate healthy increases in testosterone. So for this author, five years ago at 45 years of age suffering with low testosterone, the question I shared with you that I asked earlier in this book boiled down to this: "How can you control cortisol, and as a result, increase testosterone?"

As you've seen, <u>diet and exercise are the first two foundational steps to create the environment for healthy abundant testosterone to be produced</u>. In addition, there's a third factor that can naturally control aromatase, excess cortisol, and increase testosterone; in essence, a group of targeted, science-based nutritional supplements that I'm going to share with you right now.

About a decade ago, I filed a Health Claim Petition with the Food and Drug Administration (FDA) for the brain nutrient Phosphatidylserine. It was approved as a "Qualified Health Claim" and to date remains the only health claim of any kind to be approved by the FDA in the category of cognitive function. I was (and still am) passionate about this nutrient because of all the science that shows outstanding brain healthy benefits for those fortunate enough to add it to their diets.

Since then, the benefits of this one nutrient continue to grow in the scientific literature like no other. Today, we know that this nutrient provides significant brain benefits, *and* <u>helps to calm anxiety, stress and cortisol in healthy adults</u>. Briefly, allow me to show you the science behind Phosphatidylserine with a razor-sharp focus on its benefits on cortisol and testosterone in men.

Phosphatidylserine Reduces the "Stress Response," Decreases Cortisol, and Increases Testosterone

Phosphatidylserine (PS) has been shown to attenuate (reduce) the endocrine responses to exercise-induced acute stress.

When healthy men received single intravenous infusion of PS just prior to the initiation of a session of strenuous bicycle ergometry, typical exercise-induced increases in plasma adreno-corticotropin (ACTH) and cortisol concentrations (the typical exercise-induced stress response) did not occur.[346]

Oral PS also reduces the "stress response" to exercise or psychological stress. As examples, daily supplementation with 300 mg of PS for 1 month,[347] 400 mg for 21 days,[347] 600 mg for 21 days,[348] 800 mg for 10 days,[349] 800 mg for 21 days[348] or 800 mg for 14 days[350] suppressed the spikes in the serum concentrations of ACTH and cortisol that accompanied the initiation of cycling exercise in healthy young physically-conditioned men,[349-351] and that followed exposure to acute psychological stress in healthy young men and women.[347,348]

In the double-blind randomized placebo-controlled trial that grabbed my attention five years ago, healthy untrained young men supplemented their diets with either placebo or PS (600 mg daily).[352] After ten days of supplementation, the men participated in an exercise trial consisting of moderately-intense cycling on a stationary cycle ergometer for 5 consecutive 3-minute intervals at increasing workloads of 65%, 70%, 75%, 80% and 85% of each man's previously determined VO2max.

Compared to the lack of effect of placebo, 10 days of dietary supplementation with PS significantly suppressed the cycling-induced elevations in serum cortisol concentrations that were apparent in the men in the placebo group. In addition, take a look at this: Pre-exercise serum *total testosterone concentrations were on average 37% greater*, and pre-exercise serum *cortisol concentrations were on average 35% lower*, after just 10 days of PS supplementation.

Together these findings[346-352] indicate that supplemental PS interacts with neuronal cell membranes within the human brain to blunt the pituitary ACTH secretory response to hypothalamic stimuli, attenuating (reducing) the secretion of cortisol at rest and during and after exercise,[353] and releasing the testicular Leydig cells from cortisolemic inhibition of testosterone synthesis and secretion. In addition of course, above I pointed out that daily dietary supplementation with PS is associated with increased testosterone secretion at rest (i.e. wake up in the morning with higher testosterone).[352]

In summary, and based on the benefits stated above, take 300 mg PS with lunch and dinner (600 mg/day of PS).

Astaxanthin:
A Premier Antioxidant Powerhouse

Astaxanthin is a red carotenoid pigment belonging to the xanthophyll class of carotenoids and is found in salmon, crabs, and shrimp. Astaxanthin exhibits free radical quenching potency that is double that of beta-carotene,[354-358] about 100-fold greater than the antioxidant potency of vitamin E, [356-358] and approximately 6000 times the potency of vitamin C.[357]

Oral astaxanthin (5 mg) produces significant increases in the plasma astaxanthin concentration within one hour in men and women,[390] and is potently physiologically active unlike any other antioxidant I've ever seen. For example, adolescent male soccer players exhibited significantly increased serum antioxidant capacity after 90 days of daily dietary supplementation with just 4 mg/day of astaxanthin.[387]

After supplementing their diets for 3 weeks[390] or 12 weeks[391] with 20 mg of astaxanthin daily, 2 groups of overweight and obese men and women exhibited significant reductions in the plasma concentrations of whole-body cellular lipid peroxidation,[390,391] and significant increases in measured total circulating antioxidant capacity. Together these data indicate that astaxanthin supplementation reduced the level of oxidative stress throughout the body. To date, science shows that astaxanthin is a powerful biological antioxidant within the human body[354-396]

In summary, and for the many benefits stated above, take 4 – 6 mg of Astaxanthin twice a day (8 – 12 mg/day).

The Amazing Pomegranate: Potent Antioxidant and Anti-Aromatase Activity

Pomegranate juice, fruit, peels, seeds and oil, and their extracts, contain a large number of phytonutrient compounds, especially punicalagins and hydrolyzable ellagitannins.[397-401] Most punicalagins and ellagitannin metabolites enter the digestive system, where microbial enzymes convert them into a number of smaller ultra-active "urolithin" metabolites that pack a potent antioxidant and anti-aromatase punch. [397,403,405-407]

In a comprehensive comparative laboratory examination of relative antioxidant potency compared to red wine and nonalcoholic unfermented red grape juice, pomegranate juice exhibited an average of 2.5 times the equivalent antioxidant capacity and twice the ability to inhibit the oxidation of LDL particles by peroxides.[417] In other studies, pomegranate juice exhibited 2 to 3.5 times the antioxidant capacity of red wine or green tea,[399,420] and demonstrated more potent free radical scavenging ability than juices from grapes, cranberries, plums, kiwifruit, oranges, grapefruits, apples, pineapples, peaches or pears.[422]

Anti-Aromatase Benefits

Aromatase complex inhibition associated with pomegranate phytonutrients suggests that the consumption of these compounds should increase systemic and local tissue testosterone to estradiol ratios.[454] In fact, the publicly available scientific evidence shows that pomegranate juice and extracts are "strong" inhibitors of aromatase,[404,456] and by inhibiting aromatase, pomegranate juice and extracts can contribute to the maintenance of healthy circulating testosterone and estradiol concentrations.[454,455]

To date, the publicly available scientific evidence shows:

- Pomegranate juice, extracts and purified components of extracts are powerful antioxidants.[397-418,420-427,430-433,435,443,445-451]

- Consuming pomegranate juice or extracts increases both the circulating and endogenous antioxidant capacity in humans.[397,408,411,420,435,443,446-451,471,486,487,489,500,501]

- Pomegranate juice and extracts protect both low-density lipoproteins (LDL) and high-density lipoproteins (HDL) from oxidation.[408,424,428,435,446-452,475,478,500,501]

- Pomegranate juice and extracts reduce the level of oxidative stress throughout the body.[397,408,411,420-428,435,443,446]

In summary, and for the many benefits stated above, take 400 – 500 mg pomegranate extract twice a day (800 – 1,000 mg/day).

7

CHAPTER 7

Testosterone and Prostate Health:

In the late 1990's and potentially into mid 2000 doctors were concerned that higher healthy testosterone status might predispose a man to the development of prostate disease. Even today, some doctors recommended against increasing testosterone levels in men despite the fact that their assumptions about higher testosterone levels and its relation to prostate health does not stand up to scrutiny – at least not in science.

What's amazing is this misinformation still exists in spite of the obvious. As examples, testosterone levels are high in young men who don't have prostate disease, but low in older men, who typically do have prostate disease. That alone should make you curious. But add to that the many facts that were detailed and referenced in the beginning of this book: low testosterone is associated with increased abdominal fat, loss of insulin sensitivity, atherosclerosis, heart disease, an increased risk of cancer and many other serious quality of life issues.

Even more, numerous previously referenced studies document the positive role testosterone plays in maintaining youthful metabolic processes throughout the brain and body – and increasing testosterone eliminates the aforementioned quality of life issues. So what's going on? To answer that question, we need to again dive into the publically available science.

What Factors Cause Prostate Disease?

A major factor is: *Inflammation*. Prostate disease sets in when pathologic changes within the prostate gland result from the hyper-proliferation (high rate of cell division) of cells located predominantly in the peripheral zone of the prostate gland.[502-504] This hyper-proliferation in the periphery of the prostate gland frequently is associated with evidence of existing chronic inflammation.[502-505]

Whatever its etiologic factors may be, if left unchecked, chronic inflammation of the prostate can progress to proliferative inflammatory atrophy (PIA) of the prostate.[502-505] PIA is characterized by inflammatory cell infiltration and upregulation of cell expression of pro-inflammatory cyclooxygenase-2 (COX-2).[504-513]

Taken together, these observations have become the basis for the conclusion that inflammation of the prostate gland may sensitize prostate tissue to stimuli that can initiate dysplasia, carcinogenesis and transformation to end-stage metastatic prostate carcinoma (cancer).[502-504]

In summary:

Hyper-proliferation of the prostate gland frequently is associated with evidence of preceding or concurrent chronic inflammation.[502-505]

Inflammatory epithelial proliferation in the prostate gland can progress through several stages to become metastatic malignant prostate carcinoma.[502-513]

All this translates to the fact that "inflammation" is a potential major underlying factor or cause of prostate disease and left unchecked, serves to set up the pathologic changes that begin to manifest as prostate disease.

The Answer To Inflammation is…. Healthy Testosterone

Testosterone appears to support healthy regulation of the human immune and inflammatory systems.[33-37] In the cross-sectional observational Boston Area Community Health (BACH) survey of men aged 30 to 79 years residing in the Boston area, serum total testosterone and free testosterone concentrations were inversely correlated with plasma concentration of C-reactive protein (CRP),[33] a plasma protein that is secreted during inflammation and that participates in and stimulates the activation of immune system defense responses. In addition, a persistently elevated plasma CRP concentration is reflective of an elevated degree of chronic systemic inflammation.[34] Among a cohort of men with confirmed coronary artery disease, the plasma CRP concentration was inversely correlated with the serum free testosterone concentration.[35] In a case-control study of young men with serum total testosterone concentrations between 87 ng/dl and 750 ng/dl, serum total testosterone concentration was inversely correlated with the plasma concentrations of the pro-inflammatory cytokines, tumor necrosis factor-α (TNF-α) and macrophage inflammatory proteins 1α and 1β (MIP1α and MIP1β).[36]

Oxidative Stress and Prostate Disease

Another major factor is: *Oxidative stress*. You likely are familiar with this subject commonly referred to as "free radicals" or reactive oxygen species (ROS). By any term, science has well established that oxidative stress presents global challenges to the equilibrium, health and viability of all mammalian cells.[514] All human tissues are vulnerable to the ravages of oxidation, and the prostate gland is no exception. A byproduct of mammalian oxidative metabolism is the generation of a potent brand of reactive oxygen species (ROS) known as the "hydroxyl radical." This particular ROS can damage virtually all types of macromolecules: carbohydrates, nucleic acids (causing mutations), lipids (causing lipid peroxidation) and amino acids.

ROS both directly and indirectly produce oxidative damage to cellular constituents, including cellular DNA.[515-542] Perhaps most importantly, highly reactive intermediates of oxygen reduction (again: ROS) can react with DNA or the backbone of DNA within the cell nucleus to produce mutagenic or carcinogenic DNA adducts, and / or react with pre-existing DNA adducts to further produce pro-carcinogenic oxidized DNA adducts.[514,525-530]

Interestingly, to "add fuel to the fire" the presence of chronic inflammation further increases the local production of these DNA adducts.[537,538] And don't miss this: The prevalence of mutagenic oxidative lesions in prostate tissue DNA that are typical of those induced by hydroxyl radicals is significantly increased in cancerous prostate tissue and is significantly correlated with the extent of carcinogenic change.[540,541]

All of this translates to the fact that a deficiency of antioxidant defense is squarely implicated in the pathogenesis of prostate abnormalities, from chronic inflammation to cancer.

Antioxidants To The Rescue

Within the cells of the human prostate gland, protective intracellular enzymes are intended to catalyze the reductive conversion of ROS to less reactive compounds and prevent ROS-induced formation of DNA adducts.[504] These protective enzymes include catalase, superoxide dismutase, glutathione peroxidase, glutathione reductase and the glutathione *S*-transferase superfamily.[542]

It's critical to recognize that each of the antioxidant enzymes listed above *are built from the antioxidants and nutrients in the food that you eat.* This is another reason why an "antioxidant rich diet" is so important for optimal prostate health. As an example, just a few pages previously you learned that: "Consuming pomegranate juice or extracts increases both the circulating and endogenous antioxidant capacity in humans." The protective enzymes above are in fact the "endogenous antioxidants" that pomegranate juice and extracts so effectively support and promote.

So it's impossible to overstate the importance of maintaining your antioxidant status through diet and nutrition. I say this because experimental evidence suggests that oxidative damage to prostate cell DNA is closely associated with the initiation of benign prostatic hyperplasia (BPH) and its progression to cancer[540] and that the risk for prostate cancer is proportional to the extent of unrepaired oxidative change within DNA.[543]

Testosterone and Prostate Health

As communicated in the introduction of this chapter, in the past doctors were concerned that higher healthy testosterone status might predispose a man to the development of prostate disease and I stated that those assumptions do not stand up to scrutiny. Here's what the science says: In essence, testosterone has no impact on prostate health in adult men, at any age, in the absence of pre-existing prostate cancer.[12,455,544-564]

As examples, in peripubescent boys,[552] young men[553] and men aged 60 years and older,[455,553] pharmacologic inhibition of aromatase produced large increases in serum total and free testosterone concentrations without producing any evidence of prostate-related adverse reactions.[552,553,557]

In a case-control study in Maryland, the risk of developing prostate cancer was not related to the serum concentrations of total testosterone.[555] In a case-control study nested within the Carotene and Retinol Efficacy Trial (CARET), the risk for the development of prostate cancer was not affected by the serum concentrations of total testosterone, free testosterone, androstenedione, dehydroepiandrosterone sulfate (DHEAS), or 3α-androstenediol.[556] In the Dutch-Japanese Case Control Study on Prostate Cancer, the serum total <u>testosterone concentration did not differ</u> between men with no evidence of prostate disease, men with benign prostate hyperplasia, focal prostatic carcinoma or prostatic carcinoma.[557] In one uncontrolled clinical trial, men with symptoms suggestive of androgen deficiency received oral testosterone, 80 mg or 120 mg daily, for 6 months.[558] At the end of the trial, despite 100% to 200% increases in serum total testosterone concentrations, <u>average prostate volume and average serum prostate-specific antigen (PSA) concentration were halved</u>.

Reviewers have concluded that no study or review has shown that androgen replacement therapy (with the accompanying increase in serum androgen concentrations) is a risk factor for incident prostate cancer,[559] that there is no evidence that increasing a man's serum total testosterone concentration increases the risk of prostate cancer or benign prostate hyperplasia,[12] that there is no good evidence that increasing a man's serum total testosterone concentration will trigger the conversion of subclinical prostate cancer into clinically detectable prostate cancer,[12] that high levels of circulating endogenous testosterone have not been associated with an increased risk of prostate cancer,[560] that there is no evidence to implicate testosterone as a cause of prostate cancer, although there is flimsy evidence suggesting that testosterone may exacerbate an existing prostate cancer,[561] that circulating concentrations of total testosterone, free testosterone, DHT, androstenedione, androstenediol, DHEAS, sex hormone binding globulin, prolactin or luteinizing hormone are not associated with the risk of developing prostate cancer[562] and that there never has been a scientific basis for the contention that testosterone stimulates the unrestrained proliferation of prostate epithelial cells.[563]

A meta-analysis (a statistical analysis of several separate but similar studies) of the results of previously published studies demonstrated that the risk for developing prostate cancer is independent of the serum concentrations of total testosterone, bioavailable testosterone, DHT, androstenedione, androstenediol, DHEAS, sex hormone binding globulin, prolactin or luteinizing hormone.[564] Another meta-analysis of the results of previously published studies (performed by the Endogenous Hormones and Prostate Cancer Collaborative Group) demonstrated that the risk for developing prostate cancer is independent of the serum concentrations of total testosterone, bioavailable testosterone, DHT, androstenedione, androstenediol, DHEAS, or sex hormone binding globulin.[565] These conclusions were not changed after subanalyses according to disease severity, tumor grade, age at cancer diagnosis, year of cancer diagnosis, years since cancer diagnosis or serum prostate-specific antigen concentration. A meta-analysis of the results of 51 previously published double-blind, randomized placebo-controlled trials concluded that testosterone replacement therapy has no detrimental effect on prostate health.[566]

In joint statements released in 2010[567] and 2013,[568] the International Endocrine Aspects of Male Sexual Dysfunctions Committee and the Endocrine Subcommittee of the Standards Committee of the International Society for Sexual Medicine concluded that increasing circulating testosterone concentrations with exogenous testosterone has no effect on the risk for the development of prostate cancer, the progression of prostate cancer, the appearance of prostate-related symptoms, the development of benign prostate hyperplasia or the serum prostate-specific antigen concentration.

The publicly available scientific evidence shows:
Testosterone has no impact on prostate health in adult men, at any age, in the absence of pre-existing prostate cancer.[12,544-564,567-569]

Increasing the circulating concentration of testosterone has no effect on the risk for the development of prostate cancer, the progression of prostate cancer, the appearance of prostate-related symptoms, the development of benign prostate hyperplasia or the serum prostate-specific antigen concentration.[566-568]

8

CHAPTER 8

The Testosterone Switch Summary:

Before beginning the program, I recommend you visit with your favorite healthcare practitioner and make sure this program is for you. During that visit, get a baseline physical including your baseline Total Testosterone, Free Testosterone, DHEAS and Estradiol levels. Then give all 3-steps of this protocol your best 100% effort while setting a goal of reaching 650 – 750 ng/dL for Total Testosterone. After 30-days, go to your healthcare practitioner and retest your Total Testosterone, Free Testosterone, DHEAS and Estradiol.

An excellent resource for testing and retests is www.DirectLabs. com. A doctor's referral is not necessary at directlabs.com. Just simply use a credit card, and follow the directions to the closest LabCorp® destination near you.

After you have established your beginning levels of the 4-hormones listed above, engage the following 3-steps with a 100% effort for 30 days…

Step #1: Eat A Low Glycemic Antioxidant Rich Diet To Build Testosterone

Testosterone and insulin status are inversely correlated. This means it's important to keep insulin levels low so testosterone will remain high. Eating low glycemic foods set the stage for healthy testosterone.

Emerging research suggests healthy testosterone is tied into the healthy antioxidant status of Leydig cells in the testes. Thus, significantly increasing consumption of dietary antioxidants and nutritional supplements that deliver potent antioxidant protection from free radicals is another key to increasing healthy testosterone.

Step #2: Exercise With Intensity To Powerfully Boost Testosterone

The immediate effects of one bout of intense exercise will improve insulin, glucose homeostasis, the "stress response," and improves rates of hormone synthesis and secretion ultimately increasing testosterone.

A warm up, followed by ten 10 to 15-minutes of <u>intense exercise</u> in the form of Interval Training is all that's needed to produce a healthy hormone response.

Interval Training is: A single bout of high intensity exercise (could be cycling, sprints, stair stepper, jump squats, swimming, or my favorite: a cross-crawl Versa-Climber®) <u>to exhaustion or near-exhaustion</u>, followed by a thirty-second to one-minute recovery. Then repeat for approximately 5 to 8 sets of total intervals.

Step #3: Nutritional Supplements Can Help Control Cortisol, Aromatase, and Oxidative Stress to Build Testosterone

- 300 mg Phosphatidylserine with lunch and dinner (600 mg/day of PS).

- 4 – 6 mg of Astaxanthin twice a day (8 – 12 mg/day).

- 400 – 500 mg Pomegranate extract twice a day (800 – 1,000 mg/day).

Again: At the end of 30 days of your 100% full-tilt effort with all three (3) Testosterone Switch steps, retest by going to your healthcare practitioner or go to www.DirectLabs.com and determine your post levels of Testosterone, Free Testosterone, DHEAS and Estradiol.

Empowered with your "before and after" information, please go to www.TestosteroneSwitch.com and share your results! In addition, *please feel free to tell every man you know above the age of 30 about this program and all the benefits it has brought into your life!*

Ref.

REFERENCES

1.   http://www.lef.org/magazine/mag2010/jun2010

2.   http://abcnews.go.com/Health/Healthday/ story?id=4508669

3.   http://censusscope.org/us/chart_age.html

4.   Araujo AB, Esche GR, Kupelian V, O'Donnell AB, Travison TG, Williams RE, Clark RV, McKinlay JB. Prevalence of symptomatic androgen deficiency in men. J Clin Endocrinol Metab. 2007 Nov;92(11):4241-7.

5.   Bhasin S, Cunningham GR, Hayes FJ, Matsumoto AM, Snyder PJ, Swerdloff RS, Montori VM; Task Force, Endocrine Society. Testosterone therapy in men with androgen deficiency syndromes: An Endocrine Society clinical practice guideline. J Clin Endocrinol Metab 2010;95:2536-2559.

6.   Yeap BB, Hyde Z, Norman PE, Chubb SA, Golledge J. Associations of total testosterone, sex hormone-binding globulin, calculated free testosterone, and luteinizing hormone with prevalence of abdominal aortic aneurysm in older men. J Clin Endocrinol Metab 2010;95:1123-1130.

7.   Seftel AD, Mack RJ, Secrest AR, Smith TM. Restorative increases in serum testosterone levels are significantly correlated to improvements in sexual functioning. J

Androl 2004;25:963-972.

8.   Martinez-Jabaloyas JM, Queipo-Zaragoza A, Pastor-Hernandez F, Gil-Salom M, Chuan-Nuez P. Testosterone levels in men with erectile dysfunction. BJU Int 2006;97:1278-1283.

9.   Gray PB, Singh AB, Woodhouse LJ, Storer TW, Casaburi R, Dzekov J, Dzekov C, Sinha-Hikim I, Bhasin S. Dose-dependent effects of testosterone on sexual function, mood, and visuospatial cognition in older men. J Clin Endocrinol Metab 2005;90:3838-3846.

10. Greco EA, Spera G, Aversa A. Combining testosterone and PDE5 inhibitors in erectile dysfunction: Basic rationale and clinical evidences. Eur Urol 2006;50:940-947.

11. Zitzmann M, Faber S, Nieschlag E. Association of specific symptoms and metabolic risks with serum testosterone in older men. J Clin Endocrinol Metab 2006; doi:10.1210/jc.2006-0401.

12. Bassil N, Alkaade S, Morley JE. The benefits and risks of testosterone replacement therapy: A review. Ther Clin Risk Manag 2009;5:427-448.

13. Bassil N, Alkaade S, Morley JE. The benefits and risks of testosterone replacement therapy: A review. Ther Clin Risk Manag 2009;5:427-448.

14. Baba K, Yajima M, Carrier S, Morgan DM, Nunes L, Lue TF, Iwamoto T. Delayed testosterone replacement restores nitric oxide synthase-containing nerve fibres and the erectile response in rat penis. BJU Int

2000;85:953-958.

15. Marin R, Escrig A, Abreu P, Mas M. Androgen-dependent nitric oxide release in rat penis correlates with levels of constitutive nitric oxide synthase isoenzymes. Biol Reprod 1999;61:1012-1016.

16. Mills TM, Lewis RW, Stopper VS. Androgenic maintenance of inflow and veno- occlusion during erection in the rat. Biol Reprod 1998;59:1413-1418.

17. Park KH, Kim SW, Kim KD, Paick JS. Effects of androgens on the expression of nitric oxide synthase mRNAs in rat corpus cavernosum. BJU Int 1999;83:327-333.

18. Goglia L, Tosi V, Sanchez AM, Flamini MI, Fu XD, Zullino S, Genazzani AR, Simoncini T. Endothelial regulation of eNOS, PAI-1 and t-PA by testosterone and dihydrotestosterone in vitro and in vivo. Mol Hum Reprod 2010;16:761-769.

19. Dean RC, Lue TF. Physiology of penile erection and pathophysiology of erectile dysfunction. Urol Clin North Am 2005;32:379-395.

    Castela A, Vendeira P, Costa C. Testosterone, endothelial health, and erectile function. ISRN Endocrinol 2011;2011:839149 (doi: 10.5402/2011/839149).

20. Mills TM, Wiedmeier VT, Stopper VS. Androgen maintenance of erectile function in the rat penis. Biol Reprod 1992;46:342-348.

21. Laughlin GA, Barrett-Connor E, Bergstrom J. Low

serum testosterone and mortality in older men. J Clin Endocrinol Metab 2008;93:68-75.

22. Lehtonen A, Huupponen R, Tuomilehto J, Lavonius S, Arve S, Isoaho H, Huhtaniemi I, Tilvis R. Serum testosterone but not leptin predicts mortality in elderly men. Age Ageing 2008;37:461-464.

23. Hyde Z, Norman PE, Flicker L, Hankey GJ, Almeida OP, McCaul KA, Chubb SA, Yeap BB. Low free testosterone predicts mortality from cardiovascular disease but not other causes: The Health in Men Study. J Clin Endocrinol Metab 2012;97:179- 189.

24. Jankowska EA, Rozentryt P, Ponikowska B, Hartmann O, Kustrzycka-Kratochwil D, Reczuch K, Nowak J, Borodulin-Nadzieja L, Polonski L, Banasiak W, Poole- Wilson PA, Anker SD, Ponikowski P. Circulating estradiol and mortality in men with systolic chronic heart failure. JAMA 2009;301:1892-1901.

25. Malkin CJ, Pugh PJ, Morris PD, Asif S, Jones TH, Channer KS. Low serum testosterone and increased mortality in men with coronary heart disease. Heart 2010;96:1821-1825.

26. Tivesten A, Vandenput L, Labrie F, Karlsson MK, Ljunggren O, Mellström D, Ohlsson C. Low serum testosterone and estradiol predict mortality in elderly men. J Clin Endocrinol Metab 2009;94:2482-2488.

27. Ohlsson C, Barrett-Connor E, Bhasin S, Orwoll E, Labrie F, Karlsson MK, Ljunggren O, Vandenput L, Mellström D, Tivesten A. High serum testosterone is

associated with reduced risk of cardiovascular events in elderly men. The MrOS (Osteoporotic Fractures in Men) study in Sweden. J Am Coll Cardiol 2011;58:1674-1681.

28. Khaw KT, Dowsett M, Folkerd E, Bingham S, Wareham N, Luben R, Welch A, Day N. Endogenous testosterone and mortality due to all causes, cardiovascular disease, and cancer in men: European prospective investigation into cancer in Norfolk (EPIC-Norfolk) Prospective Population Study. Circulation 2007;116:2694-2701.

29. Araujo AB, Dixon JM, Suarez EA, Murad MH, Guey LT, Wittert GA. Clinical review: Endogenous testosterone and mortality in men: A systematic review and meta-analysis. J Clin Endocrinol Metab 2011;96:3007-3019.

30. Yeap BB, Hyde Z, Almeida OP, Norman PE, Chubb SA, Jamrozik K, Flicker L, Hankey GJ. Lower testosterone levels predict incident stroke and transient ischemic attack in older men. J Clin Endocrinol Metab 2009;94:2353-2359.

31. Moffat SD, Zonderman AB, Metter EJ, Blackman MR, Harman SM, Resnick SM. Longitudinal assessment of serum free testosterone concentration predicts memory performance and cognitive status in elderly men. J Clin Endocrinol Metab 2002;87:5001-5007.

32. Almeida OP, Yeap BB, Hankey GJ, Jamrozik K, Flicker L. Low free testosterone concentration as a poten-

tially treatable cause of depressive symptoms in older men. Arch Gen Psychiatry 2008;65:283-289.

33. Kupelian V, Chiu GR, Araujo AB, Williams RE, Clark RV, McKinlay JB. Association of sex hormones and C-reactive protein levels in men. Clin Endocrinol 2010;72:527-533.

34. Black S, Kushner I, Samols D. C-reactive protein. J Biol Chem 2004;279:48487- 48490.

35. Helaly MA, Daoud E, El-Mashad N. Does the serum testosterone level have a relation to coronary artery disease in elderly men? Curr Gerontol Geriatr Res 2011;2011:791765.

36. Bobjer J, Katrinaki M, Tsatsanis C, Lundberg Giwercman Y, Giwercman A. Negative association between testosterone concentration and inflammatory markers in young men: A nested cross-sectional study. PLoS One 2013;8:e61466 (doi: 10.1371/journal.pone.0061466).

37. Kim S, Kwon H, Park JH, Cho B, Kim D, Oh SW, Lee CM, Choi HC. A low level of serum total testosterone is independently associated with nonalcoholic fatty liver disease. BMC Gastroenterol 2012;12:69 (doi: 10.1186/1471-230X-12-69).

38. Morales A, Collier CP, Clark AF. A critical appraisal of accuracy and cost of laboratory methodologies for the diagnosis of hypogonadism: The role of free testosterone assays. Can J Urol 2012;19:6314-6318.

39. Bhasin S, Pencina M, Jasuja GK, Travison TG, Coviello

A, Orwoll E, Wang PY, Nielson C, Wu F, Tajar A, Labrie F, Vesper H, Zhang A, Ulloor J, Singh R, D'Agostino R, Vasan RS. Reference ranges for testosterone in men generated using liquid chromatography tandem mass spectrometry in a community-based sample of healthy nonobese young men in the Framingham Heart Study and applied to three geographically distinct cohorts. J Clin Endocrinol Metab 2011;96:2430-2439.

40. Nehra A, Jackson G, Miner M, Billups KL, Burnett AL, Buvat J, Carson CC, Cunningham GR, Ganz P, Goldstein I, Guay AT, Hackett G, Kloner RA, Kostis J, Montorsi P, Ramsey M, Rosen R, Sadovsky R, Seftel AD, Shabsigh R, Vlachopoulos C, Wu FC. The Princeton III Consensus recommendations for the management of erectile dysfunction and cardiovascular disease. Mayo Clin Proc 2012;87:766-778.

41. Lakshman KM, Kaplan B, Travison TG, Basaria S, Knapp PE, Singh AB, LaValley MP, Mazer NA, Bhasin S. The effects of injected testosterone dose and age on the conversion of testosterone to estradiol and dihydrotestosterone in young and older men. J Clin Endocrinol Metab 2010;95:3955-3964.

42. Srilatha B, Adaikan PG, Chong YS. Relevance of oestradiol-testosterone balance in erectile dysfunction patients' prognosis. Singapore Med J 2007;48:114-118.

43. Orrego JJ, Dimaraki E, Symons K, Barkan AL. Physiological testosterone replenishment in healthy elderly

men does not normalize pituitary growth hormone output: Evidence against the connection between senile hypogonadism and somatopause. J Clin Endocrinol Metab 2004;89:3255-3260.

44. Lamberts SW, van den Beld AW, van der Lely AJ. The endocrinology of aging. Science 1997;278:419-424.

45. Simon D, Preziosi P, Barrett-Connor E, Roger M, Saint-Paul M, Nahoul K, Papoz L. The influence of aging on plasma sex hormones in men: The Telecom Study. Am J Epidemiol 1992;135:783-791.

46. Harman SM. Testosterone, sexuality and erectile function in aging men. J Androl 2003;24:S42-S45.

47. Yeap BB, Almeida OP, Hyde Z, Norman PE, Chubb SA, Jamrozik K, Flicker L. In men older than 70 years, total testosterone remains stable while free testosterone declines with age. The Health in Men Study. Eur J Endocrinol 2007;156:585-594.

48. Kaufman JM, Vermeulen A. The decline of androgen levels in elderly men and its clinical and therapeutic implications. Endocr Rev 2005;26:833-876.

49. Orwoll E, Lambert LC, Marshall LM, Phipps K, Blank J, Barrett-Connor E, Cauley J, Ensrud K, Cummings S. Testosterone and estradiol among older men. J Clin Endocrinol Metab 2006;91:1336-1344.

50. Nakhai Pour HR, Grobbee DE, Muller M, Emmelot-Vonk M, van der Schouw YT. Serum sex hormone and plasma homocysteine levels in middle-aged and

elderly men. Eur J Endocrinol 2006;155:887-893.

51. Giton F, Urien S, Born C, Tichet J, Guéchot J, Callebert J, Bronsard F, Raynaud JP, Fiet J. Determination of bioavailable testosterone [non sex hormone binding globulin (SHBG)-bound testosterone] in a population of healthy French men: Influence of androstenediol on testosterone binding to SHBG. Clin Chem 2007;53:2160-2168.

52. Andersson AM, Jensen TK, Juul A, Petersen JH, Jørgensen T, Skakkebaek NE. Secular decline in male testosterone and sex hormone binding globulin serum levels in Danish population surveys. J Clin Endocrinol Metab 2007;92:4696-4705.

53. Travison TG, Araujo AB, Kupelian V, O'Donnell AB, McKinlay JB. The relative contributions of aging, health, and lifestyle factors to serum testosterone decline in men. J Clin Endocrinol Metab 2007;92:549-555.

54. Déchaud H, Denuzière A, Rinaldi S, Bocquet J, Lejeune H, Pugeat M. Age- associated discrepancy between measured and calculated bioavailable testosterone in men. Clin Chem 2007;53:723-728.

55. LeBlanc ES, Wang PY, Lee CG, Barrett-Connor E, Cauley JA, Hoffman AR, Laughlin GA, Marshall LM, Orwoll ES. Higher testosterone levels are associated with less loss of lean body mass in older men. J

Clin Endocrinol Metab 2011;96:3855-3863.

56. Alvarado LC. Do evolutionary life-history trade-offs influence prostate cancer risk? A review of population variation in testosterone levels and prostate cancer disparities. Evol Appl 2013;6:117-133.

57. Ferrini RL, Barrett-Connor E. Sex hormones and age: A cross-sectional study of testosterone and estradiol and their bioavailable fractions in community-dwelling men. Am J Epidemiol 1998;147:750-754.

58. Harman SM, Metter EJ, Tobin JD, Pearson J, Blackman MR; Baltimore Longitudinal Study of Aging. Longitudinal effects of aging on serum total and free testosterone levels in healthy men. Baltimore Longitudinal Study of Aging. J Clin Endocrinol Metab 2001;86:724-731.

59. Liao M, Huang X, Gao Y, Tan A, Lu Z, Wu C, Zhang Y, Yang X, Zhang H, Qin X, Mo Z. Testosterone is associated with erectile dysfunction: A cross-sectional study in Chinese men. PLoS One 2012;7:e39234 (doi: 10.1371/journal.pone.0039234).

60. Zmuda JM, Cauley JA, Kriska A, Glynn NW, Gutai JP, Kuller LH. Longitudinal relation between endogenous testosterone and cardiovascular disease risk factors in middle-aged men. A 13-year follow-up of former Multiple Risk Factor Intervention Trial participants. Am J Epidemiol 1997;146:609-617.

61. Dhindsa S, Furlanetto R, Vora M, Ghanim H, Chaudhuri A, Dandona P. Low estradiol concentrations in

men with subnormal testosterone concentrations and type 2 diabetes. Diabetes Care 2011;34:1854-1859.

62.   Feldman HA, Longcope C, Derby CA, Johannes CB, Araujo AB, Coviello AD, Bremner WJ, McKinlay JB. Age trends in the level of serum testosterone and other hormones in middle-aged men: Longitudinal results from the Massachusetts male aging study. J Clin Endocrinol Metab 2002;87:589-598.

63.   Gennari L, Merlotti D, Martini G, Gonnelli S, Franci B, Campagna S, Lucani B, Dal Canto N, Valenti R, Gennari C, Nuti R. Longitudinal association between sex hormone levels, bone loss, and bone turnover in elderly men. J Clin Endocrinol Metab 2003;88:5327-5333.

64.   Goncharov A, Rej R, Negoita S, Schymura M, Santiago-Rivera A, Morse G; Akwesasne Task Force on the Environment, Carpenter DO. Lower serum testoster-one associated with elevated polychlorinated biphenyl concentrations in Native American men. Environ Health Perspect 2009;117:1454-1160.

65.   Lapauw B, Goemaere S, Zmierczak H, Van Pottelbergh I, Mahmoud A, Taes Y, De Bacquer D, Vansteelandt S, Kaufman JM. The decline of serum testosterone levels in community-dwelling men over 70 years of age: Descriptive data and predictors of longitudinal changes. Eur J Endocrinol 2008;159:459-468.

66.   Mellström D, Johnell O, Ljunggren O, Eriksson AL, Lorentzon M, Mallmin H, Holmberg A, Redlund-

Johnell I, Orwoll E, Ohlsson C. Free testosterone is an independent predictor of BMD and prevalent fractures in elderly men: MrOS Sweden. J Bone Miner Res 2006;21:529-535.

67. Svartberg J, Midtby M, Bønaa KH, Sundsfjord J, Joakimsen RM, Jorde R. The associations of age, lifestyle factors and chronic disease with testosterone in men: The Tromsø Study. Eur J Endocrinol 2003;149:145-152.

68. Szulc P, Claustrat B, Marchand F, Delmas PD. Increased risk of falls and increased bone resorption in elderly men with partial androgen deficiency: The MINOS study. J Clin Endocrinol Metab 2003;88:5240-5247.

69. van den Beld AW, de Jong FH, Grobbee DE, Pols HA, Lamberts SW. Measures of bioavailable serum testosterone and estradiol and their relationships with muscle strength, bone density, and body composition in elderly men. J Clin Endocrinol Metab 2000;85:3276-3282.

70. Araujo AB, O'Donnell AB, Brambilla DJ, Simpson WB, Longcope C, Matsumoto AM, McKinlay JB. Prevalence and incidence of androgen deficiency in middle- aged and older men: Estimates from the Massachusetts Male Aging Study. J Clin Endocrinol Metab 2004;89:5920-5926.

71. Hak AE, Witteman JC, de Jong FH, Geerlings MI, Hofman A, Pols HA. Low levels of endogenous androgens increase the risk of atherosclerosis in elderly

men: The Rotterdam study. J Clin Endocrinol Metab 2002;87:3632-3639.

72. Strauss L, Kallio J, Desai N, Pakarinen P, Miettinen T, Gylling H, Albrecht M, Mäkelä S, Mayerhofer A, Poutanen M. Increased exposure to estrogens disturbs maturation, steroidogenesis, and cholesterol homeostasis via estrogen receptor ? in adult mouse Leydig cells. Endocrinology 2009;150:2865-2872.

73. Srilatha B, Adaikan PG. Endocrine milieu and erectile dysfunction: Is oestradiol- testosterone imbalance, a risk factor in the elderly? Asian J Androl 2011;13:569- 573.

74. Phillips GB. Relationship between serum sex hormones and glucose, insulin and lipid abnormalities in men with myocardial infarction. Proc Natl Acad Sci U S A 1977;74:1729-1733.

75. Krause DN, Duckles SP, Gonzales RJ. Local oestrogenic/ androgenic balance in the cerebral vasculature. Acta Physiol 2011;203:181-186.

76. Hu GX, Zhao BH, Chu YH, Zhou HY, Akingbemi BT, Zheng ZQ, Ge RS. Effects of genistein and equol on human and rat testicular 3?-hydroxysteroid dehydrogenase and 17?-hydroxysteroid dehydrogenase 3 activities. Asian J Androl 2010;12:519-526.

77. Kelly DM, Jones TH. Testosterone: A vascular hormone in health and disease. J Endocrinol 2013;217:R47-R71.

78. Phillips DI, Barker DJ, Fall CH, Seckl JR, Whorwood

CB, Wood PJ, Walker BR. Elevated plasma cortisol concentrations: A link between low birth weight and the insulin resistance syndrome? J Clin Endocrinol Metab 1998;83:757-760.

79. Smith GD, Ben-Shlomo Y, Beswick A, Yarnell J, Lightman S, Elwood P. Cortisol, testosterone, and coronary heart disease: Prospective evidence from the Caerphilly study. Circulation 2005;112:332-340.

80. Nielsen MF, Caumo A, Chandramouli V, Schumann WC, Cobelli C, Landau BR, Vilstrup H, Rizza RA, Schmitz O. Impaired basal glucose effectiveness but unaltered fasting glucose release and gluconeogenesis during short-term hypercortisolemia in healthy subjects. Am J Physiol Endocrinol Metab 2004;286:E102-E110.

81. Paddon-Jones D, Sheffield-Moore M, Creson DL, Sanford AP, Wolf SE, Wolfe RR, Ferrando AA. Hypercortisolemia alters muscle protein anabolism following ingestion of essential amino acids. Am J Physiol Endocrinol Metab

2003;284:E946-E953.

82. Fenske M. Role of cortisol in the ACTH-induced suppression of testicular steroidogenesis in guinea pigs. J Endocrinol 1997;154:407-414.

83. Welsh TH Jr, Bambino TH, Hsueh AJ. Mechanism of glucocorticoid-induced suppression of testicular androgen biosynthesis in vitro. Biol Reprod

1982;27:1138-1146.

84. Hu GX, Lian QQ, Lin H, Latif SA, Morris DJ, Hardy MP, Ge RS. Rapid mechanisms of glucocorticoid signaling in the Leydig cell. Steroids 2008;73:1018-1024.

85. Clark BJ, Wells J, King SR, Stocco DM. The purification, cloning, and expression of a novel luteinizing hormone-induced mitochondrial protein in MA-10 mouse Leydig tumor cells. Characterization of the steroidogenic acute regulatory protein (StAR). J Biol Chem 1994;269:28314-28322.

86. Martin LJ, Tremblay JJ. Glucocorticoids antagonize cAMP-induced Star transcription in Leydig cells through the orphan nuclear receptor NR4A1. J Mol Endocrinol 2008;41:165-175.

87. Wang X, Walsh LP, Reinhart AJ, Stocco DM. The role of arachidonic acid in steroidogenesis and steroidogenic acute regulatory (StAR) gene and protein expression. J Biol Chem 2000;275:20204-20209.

88. Gao HB, Tong MH, Hu YQ, Guo QS, Ge R, Hardy MP. Glucocorticoid induces apoptosis in rat Leydig cells. Endocrinology 2002;143:130-138.

89. McTernan PG, Anderson LA, Anwar AJ, Eggo MC, Crocker J, Barnett AH, Stewart PM, Kumar S. Glucocorticoid regulation of p450 aromatase activity in human adipose tissue: Gender and site differences. J Clin Endocrinol Metab 2002;87:1327-1336.

90. Schmidt M, Renner C, Löffler G. Progesterone in-

hibits glucocorticoid-dependent aromatase induction in human adipose fibroblasts. J Endocrinol 1998;158:401-407.

91. Simpson ER, Ackerman GE, Smith ME, Mendelson CR. Estrogen formation in stromal cells of adipose tissue of women: Induction by glucocorticosteroids. Proc Natl Acad Sci U S A 1981;78:5690-5694.

92. Wang W, Li J, Ge Y, Li W, Shu Q, Guan H, Yang K, Myatt L, Sun K. Cortisol induces aromatase expression in human placental syncytiotrophoblasts through the cAMP/Sp1 pathway. Endocrinology 2012;153:2012-2022.

93. Jezova D, Duncko R, Lassanova M, Kriska M, Moncek F. Reduction of rise in blood pressure and cortisol release during stress by Ginkgo biloba extract (EGb761) in healthy volunteers. J Physiol Pharmacol 2002;53:337-348.

94. Harbuz MS, Lightman SL. Stress and the hypothalamo-pituitary-adrenal axis: Acute, chronic and immunological activation. J Endocrinol 1992;134:327-339.

95. Lennartsson AK, Kushnir MM, Bergquist J, Billig H, Jonsdottir IH. Sex steroid levels temporarily increase in response to acute psychosocial stress in healthy men and women. Int J Psychophysiol 2012;84:246-253.

96. Leedy MG, Wilson MS. Testosterone and cortisol levels in crewmen of U.S. Air Force fighter and cargo

planes. Psychosom Med 1985;47:333-338.

97. Chatterton RT Jr, Vogelsong KM, Lu YC, Hudgens GA. Hormonal responses to psychological stress in men preparing for skydiving. J Clin Endocrinol Metab 1997;82:2503-2509.

98. Rosmond R, Dallman MF, Björntorp P. Stress-related cortisol secretion in men: Relationships with abdominal obesity and endocrine, metabolic and hemodynamic abnormalities. J Clin Endocrinol Metab 1998;83:1853-1859.

99. Choi JC, Chung MI, Lee YD. Modulation of pain sensation by stress-related testosterone and cortisol. Anaesthesia 2012;67:1146-1151.

100. Tsai EC, Matsumoto AM, Fujimoto WY, Boyko EJ. Association of bioavailable, free, and total testosterone with insulin resistance: Influence of sex hormone-binding globulin and body fat. Diabetes Care 2004;27:861-868.

101. Pitteloud N, Hardin M, Dwyer AA, Valassi E, Yialamas M, Elahi D, Hayes FJ. Increasing insulin resistance is associated with a decrease in Leydig cell testosterone secretion in men. J Clin Endocrinol Metab 2005;90:2636-2641.

102. Vikan T, Schirmer H, Njølstad I, Svartberg J. Low testosterone and sex hormone- binding globulin levels and high estradiol levels are independent predictors of type 2 diabetes in men. Eur J Endocrinol

2010;162:747-754.

103. Barrett-Connor E, Khaw KT. Endogenous sex hormones and cardiovascular disease in men. A prospective population-based study. Circulation 1988;78:539-545.

104. Simon D, Charles MA, Nahoul K, Orssaud G, Kremski J, Hully V, Joubert E, Papoz L, Eschwege E. Association between plasma total testosterone andcardiovascular risk factors in healthy adult men: The Telecom Study. J Clin Endocrinol Metab 1997;82:682-685.

105. Wickman S, Saukkonen T, Dunkel L. The role of sex steroids in the regulation of insulin sensitivity and serum lipid concentrations during male puberty: A prospective study with a P450-aromatase inhibitor. Eur J Endocrinol 2002;146:339-346.

106. Kapoor D, Goodwin E, Channer KS, Jones TH. Testosterone replacement therapy improves insulin resistance, glycaemic control, visceral adiposity and hypercholesterolaemia in hypogonadal men with type 2 diabetes. Eur J Endocrinol 2006;154:899-906.

107. Rubinow KB, Snyder CN, Amory JK, Hoofnagle AN, Page ST. Acute testosterone deprivation reduces insulin sensitivity in men. Clin Endocrinol 2012;76:281-288.

108. Kupelian V, Hayes FJ, Link CL, Rosen R, McKinlay JB. Inverse association of testosterone and the metabolic syndrome in men is consistent across race and ethnic groups. J Clin Endocrinol Metab 2008;93:3403-

3410.

109. Salehzadeh F, Rune A, Osler M, Al-Khalili L. Testosterone or 17?-estradiol exposure reveals sex-specific effects on glucose and lipid metabolism in human myotubes. J Endocrinol 2011;210:219-229.

110. Galgani J, Aguirre C, Díaz E. Acute effect of meal glycemic index and glycemic load on blood glucose and insulin responses in humans. Nutr J 2006;5:22 (doi: 10.1186/1475-2891-5-22).

111. Brand-Miller JC, Stockmann K, Atkinson F, Petocz P, Denyer G. Glycemic index, postprandial glycemia, and the shape of the curve in healthy subjects: Analysis of a database of more than 1,000 foods. Am J Clin Nutr 2009;89:97-105.

112. Esfahani A, Wong JM, Mirrahimi A, Srichaikul K, Jenkins DJ, Kendall CW. The glycemic index: Physiological significance. J Am Coll Nutr 2009;28(Suppl.):439S- 445S.

113. Jamurtas AZ, Tofas T, Fatouros I, Nikolaidis MG, Paschalis V, Yfanti C, Raptis S, Koutedakis Y. The effects of low and high glycemic index foods on exercise performance and beta-endorphin responses. J Int Soc Sports Nutr 2011;8:15 (doi: 10.1186/1550-2783-8-15).

114. Livesey G, Taylor R, Hulshof T, Howlett J. Glycemic response and health—a systematic review and meta-analysis: Relations between dietary glycemic properties and health outcomes. Am J Clin Nutr

2008;87:258S-268S.

115. Krishnan S, Newman JW, Hembrooke TA, Keim NL. Variation in metabolic responses to meal challenges differing in glycemic index in healthy women: Is it meaningful? Nutr Metab 2012;9:26 (doi: 10.1186/1743-7075-9-26).

116. Haus JM, Solomon TP, Lu L, Jesberger JA, Barkoukis H, Flask CA, Kirwan JP. Intramyocellular lipid content and insulin sensitivity are increased following a short-term low-glycemic index diet and exercise intervention. Am J Physiol Endocrinol Metab 2011;301:E511-E516.

117. Solomon TP, Haus JM, Kelly KR, Cook MD, Filion J, Rocco M, Kashyap SR, Watanabe RM, Barkoukis H, Kirwan JP. A low-glycemic index diet combined with exercise reduces insulin resistance, postprandial hyperinsulinemia, and glucose- dependent insulino-tropic polypeptide responses in obese, prediabetic humans. Am J Clin Nutr 2010;92:1359-1368.

118. Wolever TM. The glycemic index: flogging a dead horse? Diabetes Care. 1997 March;20(3):452-456.

119. Powell KF, Holt SH, Brand-Miller JC. International table of glycemic index and glycemic load values:2002. Am J of Clin Nutr. 2002;76: 5-56.

120. Committee on Military Nutrition Research, Comittee on Body Composition, Nutrition and Health. Food and Nutrition Board, Institute of Medicine: The Role of Protein and Amino Acids In Sustaining And

Enhancing Performance. National Academy Press. Washington D.C. 1999. Pp. 1-75, 85-91.

121. Garrison R. Somer E. The Nutrition Desk Reference, Third Edition. Keats Publishing, New Canaan Connecticut. 1995. 1997.

122. Laderman KA, Penny JR, Mazzucchelli F, Bresolin N, Scarlato G, Attardi G. Aging-dependent functional alterations of mitochondrial DNA (mtDNA) from human fibroblasts transferred into mtDNA-less cells. J Biol Chem 1996;271:15891-15897.

123. Wei YH, Lee HC. Oxidative stress, mitochondrial DNA mutation, and impairment of antioxidant enzymes in aging. Exp Biol Med 2002;227:671-682.

124. Dietrich MO, Horvath TL. The role of mitochondrial uncoupling proteins in lifespan. Pflugers Arch 2010;459:269-275.

125. Harman D. Free radical theory of aging: Dietary implications. Am J Clin Nutr 1972;25:839-843.

126. Harman D. The aging process. Proc Natl Acad Sci U S A 1981;78:7124-7128.

127. Ames BN, Shigenaga MK, Hagen TM. Oxidants, antioxidants, and the degenerative diseases of aging. Proc Natl Acad Sci U S A 1993;90:7915-7922.

128. Cao L, Leers-Sucheta S, Azhar S. Aging alters the functional expression of enzymatic and non-enzymatic anti-oxidant defense systems in testicular rat Leydig cells. The Journal of Steroid Biochemistry and Mo-

lecular Biology, January 2004, Pages 61–67

129. Volek JS, Kraemer WJ, Bush JA, Incledon T, Boetes M. Testosterone and cortisol in relationship to dietary nutrients and resistance exercise. J Appl Physiol 1997;82:49-54.

130. Crewther BT, Cook CJ, Gaviglio CM, Kilduff LP, Drawer S. Baseline strength can influence the ability of salivary free testosterone to predict squat and sprinting performance. J Strength Cond Res 2012;26:261-268.

131. Vingren JL, Kraemer WJ, Hatfield DL, Anderson JM, Volek JS, Ratamess NA, Thomas GA, Ho JY, Fragala MS, Maresh CM. Effect of resistance exercise on muscle steroidogenesis. J Appl Physiol 2008;105:1754-1760.

132. Hayashi Y, Nagasaka S, Takahashi N, Kusaka I, Ishibashi S, Numao S, Lee DJ, Taki Y, Ogata H, Tokuyama K, Tanaka K. A single bout of exercise at higher intensity enhances glucose effectiveness in sedentary men. J Clin Endocrinol Metab 2005;90:4035-4040.

133. Solomon TP, Haus JM, Kelly KR, Cook MD, Riccardi M, Rocco M, Kashyap SR, Barkoukis H, Kirwan JP. Randomized trial on the effects of a 7-d low-glycemic diet and exercise intervention on insulin resistance in older obese humans. Am J Clin Nutr 2009;90:1222-1229.

134. Magkos F, Mohammed BS, Mittendorfer B. Enhanced insulin sensitivity after acute exercise is not associ-

ated with changes in high-molecular weight adiponectin concentration in plasma. Eur J Endocrinol 2010b;162:61-66.

135. Magkos F, Tsekouras Y, Kavouras SA, Mittendorfer B, Sidossis LS. Improved insulin sensitivity after a single bout of exercise is curvilinearly related to exercise energy expenditure. Clin Sci 2008;114:59-64.

136. Perreault L, Lavely JM, Bergman BC, Horton TJ. Gender differences in insulin action after a single bout of exercise. J Appl Physiol 2004;97:1013-1021.

137. Rabøl R, Petersen KF, Dufour S, Flannery C, Shulman GI. Reversal of muscle insulin resistance with exercise reduces postprandial hepatic de novo lipogenesis in insulin resistant individuals. Proc Natl Acad Sci U S A 2011;108:13705-13709.

138. Hagobian TA, Sharoff CG, Stephens BR, Wade GN, Silva JE, Chipkin SR, Braun Effects of exercise on energy-regulating hormones and appetite in men and women. Am J Physiol Regul Integr Comp Physiol 2009;296:R233-R242.

139. Richards JC, Johnson TK, Kuzma JN, Lonac MC, Schweder MM, Voyles WF, Bell C. Short-term sprint interval training increases insulin sensitivity in healthy adults but does not affect the thermogenic response to ?-adrenergic stimulation. J Physiol 2010;588:2961-2972.

140. Winnick JJ, Sherman WM, Habash DL, Stout MB, Failla ML, Belury MA, Schuster DP. Short-term

aerobic exercise training in obese humans with type 2 diabetes mellitus improves whole-body insulin sensitivity through gains in peripheral, not hepatic insulin sensitivity. J Clin Endocrinol Metab 2008;93:771-778.

141. Harrison M, O'Gorman DJ, McCaffrey N, Hamilton MT, Zderic TW, Carson BP, Moyna NM. Influence of acute exercise with and without carbohydrate replacement on postprandial lipid metabolism. J Appl Physiol 2009;106:943-949.

142. Tremblay MS, Copeland JL, Van Helder W. Effect of training status and exercise mode on endogenous steroid hormones in men. J Appl Physiol 2004;96:531-539.

143. Fry AC, Kraemer WJ, Ramsey LT. Pituitary-adrenal-gonadal responses to high- intensity resistance exercise overtraining. J Appl Physiol 1998;85:2352-2359.

144. Hackney AC, Viru M, VanBruggen M, Janson T, Karelson K, Viru A. Comparison of the hormonal responses to exhaustive incremental exercise in adolescent and young adult males. Arq Bras Endocrinol Metabol 2011;55:213-218.

145. Gawel MJ, Park DM, Alaghband-Zadeh J, Rose FC. Exercise and hormonal secretion. Postgrad Med J 1979;55:373-376.

146. Kraemer WJ, Häkkinen K, Newton RU, Nindl BC, Volek JS, McCormick M, Gotshalk LA, Gordon SE, Fleck SJ, Campbell WW, Putukian M, Evans WJ.

Effects of heavy-resistance training on hormonal response patterns in younger vs. older men. J Appl Physiol 1999;87:982-992.

147. Simao R, Leite RD, Speretta GFF, Maior AS, de Salles BF, de Souza Junior TP, Vingren JL, Willardson JM. Influence of upper-body exercise order on hormonal responses in trained men. Appl Physiol Nutr Metab 2013;38:177-181.

148. Parker AG, Gordon J, Thornton A, Byars A, Lubker J, Bartlett M, Byrd M, Oliver J, Simbo S, Rasmussen C, Greenwood M, Kreider RB. The effects of IQPLUS Focus on cognitive function, mood and endocrine response before and following acute exercise. J Int Soc Sports Nutr 2011;8:16 (doi: 10.1186/1550-2783-8-16).

149. Sutton JR, Coleman MJ, Casey J, Lazarus L. Androgen responses during physical exercise. Br Med J 1973;1(5852):520-522.

150. Arazi H, Damirchi A, Asadi A. Age-related hormonal adaptations, muscle circumference and strength development with 8 weeks moderate intensity resistance training. Ann Endocrinol 2013;74:30-35.

151. Hickson RC, Hidaka K, Foster C, Falduto MT, Chatterton RT Jr. Successive time courses of strength development and steroid hormone responses to heavy-resistance training. J Appl Physiol 1994;76:663-670.

152. Black JE, Isaacs KR, Anderson BJ, Alcantara AA, Greenough WT. Learning causes synaptogenesis,

whereas motor activity causes angiogenesis, in cerebellar cortex of adult rats. Proc Natl Acad Sci USA 1990;87:5568-5572.

153. Altman J, Das GD. Autoradiographic examination of the effects of enriched environment on the rate of glial multiplication in the adult rat brain. Nature 1964;204:1161-1163.

154. Pysh JJ, Weiss GM. Exercise during development induces an increase in Purkinje cell dendritic tree size. Science 1979;206:230-232.

155. Isaacs KR, Anderson BJ, Alcantara AA, Black JE, Greenough WT. Exercise and the brain: Angiogenesis in the adult rat cerebellum after vigorous physical activity and motor skill learning. J Cerebral Blood Flow Metab 1992;12:110-119.

156. Eccles JC. An instruction-selection theory of learning in the cerebellar cortex. Brain Res 1977;127:327- 352.

157. Herholz K, Buskies B, Rist M, Pawlik G, Hollmann W, Heiss W-D. Regional cerebral blood flow in man at rest and during exercise. J Neurol 1987;234:9-13.

158. Jorgensen LG, Perko M, Hanel B, Schroeder TV, Secher NH. Middle cerebral artery flow velocity and blood flow during exercise and muscle ischemia in humans. J Appl Physiol 1992;72:1123-1132.

159. Jorgensen LG, Perko M, Secher NH. Regional cerebral artery mean velocity and blood flow during dynamic exercise in humans. J Appl Physiol 1992;73:1825-

1830.

160. Thomas SN, Schroeder T, Secher NH, Mitchell JH. Cerebral blood flow during submaximal and maximal dynamic exercise in humans. J Appl Physiol 1989;67:744-748.

161. Dustman RE, Ruhling RO, Russell EM, Shearer DE, Bonekat HW, Shigeoka JW, Wood JS, Bradford DC. Aerobic exercise training and improved neuropsychological function of older individuals. Neurobiol Aging 1984;5:35-42.

162. Offenbach SI, Chodzko-Zajko WJ, Ringel RL. The relationship between physiological status, cognition, and age in adult men. Bull Psychon Soc 1990;28:112-114.

163. Rogers RL, Meyer JS, Mortel KF. After reaching retirement age physical activity sustains cerebral perfusion and cognition. J Am Geriatr Soc 1990;38:123-128.

164. Krebs P, Eickelberg W, Krobath H, Baruch I. Effects of physical exercise on peripheral vision and learning in children with spina bifida manifesta. Percept Mot Skills 1989;68:167-174.

165. Caterino MC, Polak ED. Effects of two types of activity on the performance of second-, third-, and fourth-grade students on a test of concentration. Percept Mot Skills 1999;89:245-248.

166. Gabbard C, Barton J. Effects of physical activity on mathematical computation among young children. J

Psychol 1979;103:287-288.

167. Blomstrand E, Hassmen P, Newsholme EA. Effect of branched-chain amino acid supplementation on mental performance. Acta Physiol Scand 1991;143:225-226.

168. Gondola JC, Tuckman BW. Effects of a systematic program of exercise on selected measures of creativity. Percept Mot Skills 1985;60:53-54.

169. Hogervorst E, Riedel W, Jeukendrup A, Jolles J. Cognitive performance after strenuous physical exercise. Percept Mot Skills 1996;83:479-488.

170. Blumenthal JA, Emery CF, Madden DJ, George LK, Coleman RE, Riddle MW, McKee DC, Reasoner J, Williams RS. Cardiovascular and behavioral effects of aerobic exercise training in healthy older men and women. J Gerontol 1989;44:M147-M157.

171. Baylor AM, Spirduso WW. Systematic aerobic exercise and components of reaction time in older women. J Gerontol 1988;43:P121-P126.

172. Hascelik Z, Basgoze O, Turker K, Narman S, Ozker R. The effects of physical training on physical fitness tests and auditory and visual reaction times of volleyball players. J Sports Med 1989;29:234-239.

173. Clarkson-Smith L, Hartley AA. Structural equation models of relationships between exercise and cognitive abilities. Psychol Aging 1990;5:437-434.

174. Paffenbarger RS Jr, Lee I-M, Leung R. Physical activity

and personal characteristics associated with depression and suicide in American college men. Acta Psychiatr Scand 1994;Suppl 377:16-22.

175. Tilley AJ, Bohle P. Twisting the night away: The effects of all night disco dancing on reaction time. Percept Mot Skills 1988;66:107-112.

176. Molloy DW, Beerschoten DA, Borrie MJ, Crilly RG, Cape RDT. Acute effects of exercise on neuropsychological function in elderly subjects. J Am Geriatr Soc 1988;36:29-33.

177. Steinberg H, Sykes EA, Moss T, Lowery S, LeBoutillier N, Dewey A. Exercise enhances creativity independently of mood. Br J Sports Med 1997;31:240-245.

178. Blomquist KB, Danner F. Effects of physical conditioning on information-processing efficiency. Percept Mot Skills 1987;65:175-186.

179. Fordyce DE, Wehner JM. Physical activity enhances spatial learning performance with an associated alteration in hippocampal protein kinase C activity in C57BL/6 and DBA/2 mice. Brain Res 1993;619:111- 119.

180. Casanueva F, Villanueva L, Penalva A, Vila T, Cabezas-Cerrato J. Free fatty acid inhibition of exercise-induced growth hormone secretion. Horm Metab Res 1981;13:348-350.

181. Chang FE, Dodds WG, Sullivan M, Kim MH, Malarkey WB. The acute effects of exercise on prolactin and growth hormone secretion: comparison between

sedentary women and women runners with normal and abnormal menstrual cycles. J Clin Endocrinol Metab 1986;62:551-556.

182. Di Luigi L, Guideti L, Nordio M, Baldari C, Romanelli F. Acute effect of physical exercise on serum insulin-like growth factor-binding protein 2 and 3 in healthy men: role of exercise-linked growth hormone secretion. Int J Sports Med 2001;22:103-110.

183. Harada T, Yamauchi T, Tsukanaka A, Matsumura Y, Kurono M, Honda A, Matsui N. Involvement of mus- carinic cholinergic and alpha2-adrenergic mechanisms in growth hormone secretion during exercise in humans. Eur J Appl Physiol 2000;83:268-273.

184. Harro J, Rimm H, Harro M, Grauberg M, Karelson K, Viru AM. Association of depressiveness with blunted growth hormone response to maximal physical exercise in young healthy men. Psychoneuroendocrinology 1999;24:505-517.

185. Buckler JM. The relationship between changes in plasma growth hormone levels and body temperature occurring with exercise in man. Biomedicine 1973;19:193-197.

186. Vanhelder WP, Radomski MW, Goode RC. Growth hormone responses during intermittent weight lifting exercise in men. Eur J Appl Physiol 1984;53:31-34.

187. Sutton JR, Jones NL, Toews CJ. Growth hormone secretion in acid-base alterations at rest and during

exercise. Clin Sci Molec Med 1976;50:241-247.

188. Roth J, Glick SM, Yalow RS, Berson SA. Secretion of human growth hormone: Physiologic and experimental modification. Metabolism 1963;12:577-579.

189. Kozlowski S, Chwalbinska-Moneta J, Vigas M, Kaciuba-Uscilko H, Nazar K. Greater serum GH response to arm than to leg exercise performed at equivalent oxygen uptake. Eur J Appl Physiol 1983;52:131-135.

190. Lassarre C, Girard F, Durand J, Raynaud J. Kinetics of human growth hormone during submaximal exercise. J Appl Physiol 1974;37:826-830.

191. Sutton J, Lazarus L. Growth hormone in exercise: Comparison of physiological and pharmacological stimuli. J Appl Physiol 1976;41:523-527.

192. Vanhelder WP, Goode RC, Radomski MW. Effect of anaerobic and aerobic exercise of equal duration and work expenditure on plasma growth hormone levels. Eur J Appl Physiol 1984;52:255-257.

193. Marcell TJ, Wiswell RA. Hawkins SA, Tarpenning KM. Age-related blunting of growth hormone secretion during exercise may not be solely due to increased somatostatin tone. Metabolism 1999;48:665-670.

194. Borst SE, Millard WJ, Lowenthal DT. Growth hormone, exercise and ageing: The future of therapy for the frail elderly. J Am Geriatr Soc 1994;42:528-535.

195. Craig BW, Brown R, Everhart J. Effects of progressive resistance training on growth hormone and testos-

terone levels in young and elderly subjects. Mech Ageing Dev 1989;49:159-169.

196. Parkin JM. Exercise as a test of growth hormone secretion. Acta Endocrinol Suppl (Copenh) 1986;279:47-50.

197. Peyreigne C, Bouix D, Micallef JP, Mercier J, Bringer J, Prefaut C, Brun JF. Exercise-induced growth hormone secretion and hemorheology during exercise in elite athletes. Clin Hemorheol Microcirc 1998;19:169-176.

198. Pritzlaff CJ, Wideman L, Bkumer J, Jensen M, Abbott RD, Gaesser GA, Veldhuis JD, Weltman A. Catecholamine release, growth hormone secretion, and energy expenditure during exercise vs. recovery in men. J Appl Physiol 2000;89:937-946.

199. Bunt JC, Boileau RA, Bahr JM, Nelson RA. Sex and training differences in human growth hormone during prolonged exercise. J Appl Physiol 1986;61:1796-1801.

200. Pyka G, Taaffe DR, Marcus R. Effect of a sustained program of resistance training on the acute growth hormone response to resistance exercise in older adults. Horm Metab Res 1994;26:330-333.

201. Weltman A, Pritzlaff CJ, Wideman L, Weltman JY, Blumer JL, Abbott RD, Hartman ML, Veldhuis JD. Exercise-dependent growth hormone release is linked to markers of heightened central adrenergic out- flow.

J Appl Physiol 2000;89:629-635.

202. Brilloon D, Nabil N, Jacobs LS. Cholinergic but not serotonergic mediation of exercise-induced growth hormone secretion. Endocr Res 1986;12:137-146.

203. Weltman A, Weltman JY, Schurrer R, Evans WS, Veldhuis JD, Rogol AD. Endurance training amplifies the pulsatile release of growth hormone: Effects of training intensity. J Appl Physiol 1992;72:2188-2196.

204. Felsing NE, Brasel JA, Cooper DM. Effect of low and high intensity exercise on circulatory growth hormone in men. J Clin Endocrinol Metab 1992;75:157-162.

205. Raynaud J, Capderou A, Martineau JP, Bordachar J, Durand J. Intersubject variability in growth hormone time course during different types of work. J Appl Physiol 1983;55:1682-1687.

206. Butler RW, Dickinson WA, Katholi C, Halsey JH. The comparative effects of organic brain disease on cerebral blood flow and measured intelligence. Ann Neurol 1983;13:155-159.

207. Pritzlaff-Roy C, Widemen L, Weltman J, et al. Gender governs the relationship between exercise intensity and growth hormone release in young adults. J Appl Physiol 92: 2053-2060, 2002.

208. Pritzlaff C, Widemen L, Weltman J, et al. Impact of acute exercise intensity on pulsatile growth hormone release in men. J Appl Physiol Vol. 87, Issue 2, 498-

504, August 1999.

209. Felsing N, Brasel J, Cooper D. Effect of low and high intensity exercise on circulating growth hormone in men. Journal of Clinical Endocrinology & Metabolism, Vol 75, 157-162, 1992.

210. Cappon JP, Ipp E, Brasel JA, Cooper DM. Acute effects of high fat and high glucose meals on the growth hormone response to exercise. Clin Endocrinol Metab. 1993 Jun;76(6):1418-22.

211. Cappon J, Brasel JA, Mohan S, Cooper DM. Effect of brief exercise on circulating insulin-like growth factor I. J Appl Physiol. 1994 Jun;76(6):2490-6.

212. Kraemer WJ, Gordon SE, Fleck SJ, et al. Endogenous anabolic hormonal and growth factor responses to heavy resistance exercise in males and females. Int J Sports Med. 1991 Apr;12(2):228-35.

213. Tremblay A, Simoneau JA, Bouchard C. Impact of exercise intensity on body fatness and skeletal muscle metabolism. Metabolism. 1994 Jul;43(7):814-8.

214. Osterberg KL, Melby CL. Effect of acute resistance exercise on postexercise oxygen consumption and resting metabolic rate in young women. Int J Sport Nutr Exerc Metab. 2000 Mar;10(1):71-81.

215. Schuenke MD, Mikat RP, McBride JM. Effect of an acute period of resistance exercise on excess postexercise oxygen consumption: implications for body mass management. Eur J Appl Physiol. 2002

Mar;86(5):411-7.

216. MacDougall JD, Hicks AL, MacDonald JR, McKelvie RS, Green HJ, and Smith KM. Muscle performance and enzymatic adaptations to sprint interval training. J Appl Physiol 84: 2138-2142, 1998.

217. Ross A and Leveritt M. Long-term metabolic and skeletal muscle adaptations to short-sprint training: implications for sprint training and tapering. Sports Med 15: 1063-1082, 2001.

218. Burgomaster KA, Hughes SC, Heigenhauser GJ, Bradwell SN, Gibala MJ. Six sessions of sprint interval training increases muscle oxidative potential and cycle endurance capacity in humans. J Appl Physiol. 2005 Jun;98(6):1985-90.

219. Walsh BT, Puig-Antich J, Goetz R, Gladis M, Novacenko H, Glassman AH. Sleep and growth hormone secretion in women athletes. Electroencephalogr Clin Neurophysiol 1984;57:528-531.

220. Adamson L, Hunter WM, Ogunremi OO, Oswald I, Percy-Robb IW. Growth hormone increase during sleep after daytime exercise. J Endocrinol 1974;62:473-478.

221. King J, Panton L, Broeder C, et al. A Comparison of High Intensity vs. Low Intensity Exercise on Body Composition in Overweight Women. Medicine & Science in Sports & Exercise. 33(5) Supplement 1:S228, May 2001.

222. Sonntag WE, Hylka VW, Meites J. Growth hormone

restores protein synthesis in skeletal muscle of old male rats. J Gerontol 1985;40:684-694.

223. Crist DM, Peake GT, Loftfield RB, Kraner JC, Egan PA. Supplemental growth hormone alters body com- position, muscle protein metabolism and serum lipids in fit adults: characterization of dose-dependent and response-recovery effects. Mech Ageing Dev 1991;58:191-205.

224. Snyder DK, Underwood LE, Clemmons DR. Anabolic effects of growth hormone in obese diet-restricted subjects are dose dependent. Am J Clin Nutr 1990;52:431-437.

225. Petersen SR, Holaday NJ, Jeevanandam M. Enhancement of protein synthesis efficiency in parenterally fed trauma victims by adjuvant recombinant human growth hormone. J Trauma 1994;36:726-733.

226. De Feo P, Perriello G, Torlone E, Ventura MM, Santeusanio F, Brunetti P, Gerich JE, Bolli GB. Demonstration of a role for growth hormone in glucose counterregulation. Am J Physiol 1989;256:E835-E843.

227. Wolf RF, Heslin MJ, Newman E, Pearlstone DB, Gonenne A, Brennan MF. Growth hormone and insulin combine to improve whole-body and skeletal muscle protein kinetics. Surgery 1992;112:284-292.

228. Bazarre TL, Johanson AJ, Huseman CA, Varma MM, Blizzard RM. Human growth hormone changes with age. Excerpta Med 1975;381:261.

229. Copeland KC, Nair KS. Acute growth hormone effects

on amino acid and lipid metabolism. J Clin Endocrinol Metab 1994;78:1040-1047.

230. Keller V, Schnell H, Girard J, Stauffacher W. Effect of physiological elevation of plasma growth hor- mone levels on ketone body kinetics and lipolysis in normal acutely insulin deficient man. Diabetologia 1984;26:103-108.

231. Merimee TJ. Growth hormone: secretion and action. In: De Groot, L.J. (ed.). Endocrinology. Grune & Stratton, New York, 1979.

232. Snyder DK, Underwood LE, Clemmons DR. Persistent lipolytic effect of exogenous growth hormone during caloric restriction. Am J Med 1995;98:129-134.

233. Moller N, Moller J, Jorgensen JO, Ovesen P, Schmitz O, Alberti KG, Christiansen JS. Impact of 2 weeks high dose growth hormone treatment on basal and insulin stimulated substrate metabolism in humans. Clin Endocrinol 1993;39:577-581.

234. Vernon RG. GH inhibition of lipogenesis and stimulation of lipolysis in sheep adipose tissue: involvement of protein serine phosphorylation and dephosphorylation and phospholipase C. J Endocrinol 1996;150:129-140.

235. Piatti PM, Monti LD, Caumo A, Conti M, Magni F, Galli-Kienle M, Fochesato E, Pizzini A, Baldi L, Valsecchi G, Pontiroli AE. Mediation of the hepatic effects of growth hormone by its lipolytic activity. J

Clin Endocrinol Metab 1999;84:1658-1663.

236. Rudman D, Feller AG, Nagraj HS, Gergans GA, Lalitha PY, Goldberg AF, Schlenker RA, Cohn L, Rudman IW, Mattson DE. Effects of human growth hormone in men over 60 years old. N Engl J Med 1990;323:1-5.

237. LaFranchi S, Buist NR, Jhaveri B, Klevit H. Amino acids as substrates in children with growth hormone deficiency and hypoglycemia. Pediatrics 1981;68:260-264.

238. Sonntag WE, Forman LJ, Mikki N, Meites J. Growth hormone secretion and neuroendocrine regulation. In: CRC Handbook of Endocrinology. CRC Press, Boca Raton, FL, 1981, pp. 35-59.

239. Clemmons DR, Snyder DK, Williams R, Underwood LE. Growth hormone administration conserves lean body mass during dietary restriction in obese subjects. J Clin Endocrinol Metab 1987;64:878-883.

240. Snyder DK, Clemmons DR, Underwood LE. Treatment of obese, diet restricted subjects with growth hormone for 11 weeks: effects on anabolism, lipolysis, and body composition. J Clin Endocrinol Metab 1988;67:54-61.

241. Deijen JB, de Boer H, Blok GJ, van der Veen EA. 1996 Cognitive impairments and mood disturbances in growth hormone deficient men. Psychoneuroendocrinology. 21:313-322.

242. Deijen JB, De Boer H, Van der Veen EA. 1998 Cogni-

tive changes during growth hormone replacement in adult men. Psychoneuroendocrinology. 23:45-55.

243. Papadakis MA, Grady D, Tierney MJ, Black D, Wells L, Grunfeld, C. 1995 Insulin-like growth factor 1 and functional status in healthy older men. J Am Geriatr Soc. 43:1350-1355.

244. Mahajan T, Crown A, Checkley S, Farmer A, Lightman S. Atypical depression in growth hormone deficient adults, and the beneficial effect quality of life. Eur J Endocrinol. 2004 Sep;151(3):325-32.

245. Arwert LI, Deijen JB, Muller M, Drent ML. Long-term growth hormone treatment preserves GH-induced memory and mood improvements: a 10-year follow-up study in GH-deficient adult men. Horm Behav. 2005 Mar;47(3):343-9.

246. Kalmijn S, et al. A Prospective Study on Circulating Insulin-Like Growth Factor I (IGFI), IGF-Binding Proteins, and Cognitive Function in the Elderly. Journal of Clinical Endocrinology & Metabolism Vol. 85, No. 12 4551-4555.

247. Duke University Medical News Office: http://dukemed-news.org/news/article.php?id=119

248. Hagberg JM, Seals DR, Yerg JE, Gavin J, Gingerich R, Premachandra B, Holloszy JO. Metabolic respons- es to exercise in young and old athletes and sedentary men. J Appl Physiol 1988;65:900-908.

249. Vanhelder WP, Casey K, Goode RC, Radomski WM. Growth hormone regulation in two types of aerobic

exercise of equal oxygen uptake. Eur J Appl Physiol 1986;55:236-239.

250. Karagjorgos A, Garcia JF, Brooks GA. Growth hormone response to continuous and intermittent exercise. Med Sci Sports 1979;11:302-307.

251. Pyka G, Wiswell RA, Marcus R. Age-dependent effect of resistance exercise on growth hormone secretion in people. J Clin Endocrinol Metab 1992;75:404-407.

252. Hakkinen K, Pakarinen A. Acute hormonal responses to heavy resistance exercise in men and women at different ages. Int J Sports Med 1995;16:507-513.

253. Pyka G, Taaffe DR, Marcus R. Effect of a sustained program of resistance training on the acute growth hormone response to resistance exercise in older adults. Horm Metab Res 1994;26:330-333.

254. Anderson MF, Aberg MA, Nilsson M, Eriksson PS. Insulin-like growth factor-1 and neurogenesis in the adult mammalian brain. Brain Res Dev Brain Res 2002;134:115-122.

255. Saatman KE, Contreras PC, Smith DH, Raghupathi R, McDermott KL, Fernandez SC, Sanderson KL, Voddi M, McIntosh TK. Insulin-like growth factor-1 (IGF-1) improves both neurological motor and cognitive outcome following experimental brain injury. Exp Neurol 1997;147:418-427.

256. Guan J, Skinner SJ, Beilharz EJ, Hua KM, Hodgkinson S, Gluckman PD, Williams CE. The movement of IGF-1 into the brain parenchyma after hypoxic-

ischaemic injury. Neuro Report 1996;7:632-636.

257. Yehuda R, Fairman KR, Meyer JS. Enhanced brain cell proliferation following early adrenalectomy in rats. J Neurochem 1989;53:241-248.

258. Cameron HA, Gould E. Adult neurogenesis is regulated by adrenal steroids in the dentate gyrus. Neuroscience 1994;61:203-209.

259. Ohl F, Michaelis T, Vollmann-Honsdorf GK, Kirsch-baum C, Fuchs E. Effect of chronic psychosocial stress and long-term cortisol treatment on hippocam-pus-mediated memory and hippocampal volume: A pilot study in tree shrews. Psychoneuroendocrinology 2000;25:357-363.

260. Cameron HA, Tanapat P, Gould E. Adrenal steroids and N-methyl-D-aspartate receptor activation regulate neurogenesis in the dentate gyrus of adult rats through a common pathway. Neuroscience 1998;82:349- 354.

261. Gould E, Woolley CS, McEwen BS. Short term gluco-corticoid manipulations affect neuronal morphology and survival in the adult dentate gyrus. Neuroscience 1990;37:367-375.

262. Sloviter RS, Valiquette G, Abrams GM, Ronk EC, Sollar AL, Lam P, Neubort S. Selective loss of hippocampal granule cells in the mature rat brain after adrenalec-tomy. Science 1989;243:1432-1437.

263. Joels M, de Kloet ER. Control of neuronal excitabil-ity by corticosteroid hormones. Trends Neurosci

1992;15:25-30.

264. Pavlides C, Watanabe Y, McEwen BS. Effects of gluco-corticoids on hippocampal long-term potentiation. Hippocampus 1993;3:183-192.

265. Magarinos AM, McEwen BS. Stress-induced atrophy of apical dendrites of hippocampal CA3c neurons: Involvement of glucocorticoid secretion and excitatory amino acid receptors. Neuroscience 1995;69:88- 89.

266. Wooley CS, Gould EW, McEwen BS. Exposure to excess glucocorticoids alters dendritic morphology of adult pyramidal neurons. Brain Res 1990;531:225-231.

267. McEwen BS, Sapolsky RM. Stress and cognitive function. Curr Opin Neurobiol 1995;5:205-216.

268. Fuchs E, Flugge G, Ohl F, Lucassen P, Vollmann-Honsdorf GK, Michaelis T. Psychosocial stress, gluco-corticoids, and structural alterations in the tree shrew hippocampus. Physiol Behav 2001;73:285-291.

269. Wolf OT, Convit A, McHugh PF, Kandil E, Thorn EL, De Santi S, McEwen BS, de Leon MJ. Cortisol differentially affects memory in young and elderly men. Behav Neurosci 2001;115:1002-1011.

270. Wolf OT, Schommer NC, Hellhammer DH, McEwen BS, Kirschbaum C. The relationship between stress induced cortisol levels and memory differs between men and women. Psychoneuroendocrinology 2001;26:711-720.

271. Gurvits TV, Shenton ME, Hokama H, Ohta H, Lasko

NB, Orr SP, Kikinis R, Jolesz FA, McCarley RW, Pitman RK. Reduced hippocampal volume on magnetic resonance imaging in chronic post-traumatic stress disorder. Biol Psychiatry 1996;40:1091-1099.

272. Lupien SJ, De Leon M, De Santi S, Convit A, Tarshish C, Nair NPV, Thakur M, McEwen BS, Hauger RL, Meaney MJ. Cortisol levels during human aging predict hippocampal atrophy and memory deficits. Nature Neurosci 1998;1:69-73.

273. McEwen BS. Possible mechanisms for atrophy of the human hippocampus. Mol Psychiatry 1997;2:255-262.

274. McEwen BS. Stress and hippocampal plasticity. Ann Rev Neurosci 1999;22:105-122.

275. Steptoe A, Butler N. Sports participation and emotional well-being in adolescents. Lancet 1996;347:1789-1792.

276. Blumenthal JA, Schocken DD, Needels TL, Hindle P. Psychological and physiological effects of physical conditioning on the elderly. J Psychosom Res 1982;26:505-510.

277. Boutcher SH, Landers DM. The effects of vigorous exercise on anxiety, heart rate, and alpha activity of runners and nonrunners. Psychophysiology 1988;25:696-702.

278. Doyne EJ, Ossip-Klein DJ, Bowman ED, Osborn KM, McDougall-Wilson IB, Neimeyer RA. Running versus weight lifting in the treatment of depression. J

Consult Clin Psychol 1987;55:748-754.

279. Emery CF, Schein RL, Hauck ER, MacIntyre NR. Psychological and cognitive outcomes of a randomized trial of exercise among patients with chronic obstructive pulmonary disease. Health Psychol 1998;17:232-240.

280. Fletcher GF. How to implement physical activity in primary and secondary prevention. Circulation 1997;96:355-357.

281. Folkins CH. Effects of physical training on mood. J Clin Psychol 1976;32:385-387.

282. Fremont J, Craighead LW. Aerobic exercise and cognitive therapy in the treatment of dysphoric moods. Cognitive Ther Res 1987;11:241-251.

283. Kennedy MM, Newton M. Effect of exercise intensity on mood in step aerobics. J Sports Med Phys Fitness. 1997;37:200-204.

284. McCann IL, Holmes DS. Influence of aerobic exercise on depression. J Personality Soc Psychol 1984;46:1142-1147.

285. Moses J, Steptoe A, Matthews A, Edwards S. The effects of exercise training on mental well-being in the normal population: A controlled trial. J Psychosom Res 1989;33:47-61.

286. Norris R, Carroll D, Cochrane R. The effects of aerobic and anaerobic training on fitness, blood pressure, and psychological stress and well-being. J Psychosom Res

1990;34:367-375.

287. Nouri S, Beer J. Relations of moderate physical exercise to scores on hostility, aggression and trait-anxiety. Peceptual Motor Skills 1989;68:1191-1194.

288. Otto J. The effects of physical exercise on psycho-physiological reactions under stress. Cognition and Emotion 1990;4:341-357.

289. Partonen T, Leppamaki S, Hurme J, Lonnqvist J. Randomized trial of physical exercise alone or combined with bright light on mood and health-related quality of life. Psychol Med 1998;28:1359-1364.

290. Petruzzello SJ, Landers DM, Hatfield BD, Kubitz KA, Salazar W. A meta-analysis on the anxiety-reducing effects of acute and chronic exercise. Sports Med 1991;11:143-182.

291. Roth DL. Acute emotional and psychophysiological effects of aerobic exercise. Psychophysiology 1989;26:593-602.

292. Steptoe A, Edwards S, Moses J, Mathews A. The effects of exercise training on mood and perceived coping ability in anxious adults from the general population. J Psychosom Res 1989;33:537-547.

293. Weinberg R, Jackson A, Kolodny K. The relationship of massage and exercise to mood enhancement. The Sport Psychologist 1988;2:202-211.

294. Williams JM, Getty D. Effects of levels of exercise on psychological mood stress, physical fitness,

and plasma beta-endorphin. Percept Mot Skills 1986;63:1099-1105.

295. DasGupta K. Treatment of depression in elderly patients. Arch Fam Med 1998;7:274-280.

296. King AC, Taylor CB, Haskell WL. Effects of differing intensities and formats of 12 months of exercise train- ing on psychological outcomes in older adults. Health Psychol 1993;12:292-300.

297. Singh NA, Clements KM, Fiatarone MA. A randomized controlled trial of progressive resistance training in depressed elders. J Gerontol 1997;52:M27-M35.

298. Daniel M, Martin AD, Carter J. Opiate receptor block-ade by naltrexone and mood state after acute physi-cal activity. Br J Sports Med 1992;26:111-115.

299. Thirlaway K, Benton D. Participation in physical activ-ity and cardiovascular fitness have different effects on mental health and mood. J Psychosom Res 1992;36:657-665.

300. Wildmann J, Kruger A, Schmole M, Niemann J, Mat-thaei H. Increase of circulating b-endorphin-like immu- noreactivity correlates with the change in feeling of pleasantness after running. Life Sci 1986;38:997-1003.

301. Yeung RB. The acute effects of exercise on mood state. J Psychosom Res 1996;40:123-141.

302. Camacho TC, Roberts RE, Lazarus NB, Kaplan GA, Cohen RD. Physical activity and depression: Evi-

dence from the Alameda County Study. Am J Epidemiol 1991;134:220-231.

303. Farmer ME, Locke BZ, Moscicki EK, Dannenberg AL, Larson DB, Radloff LS. Physical activity and depressive symptoms: The NHANES I Epidemiologic Follow-up Study. Am J Epidemiol 1988;128:1340-1351.

304. Weyerer S. Physical inactivity and depression in the community. Evidence from the Upper Bavarian Field Study. Int J Sports Med 1992;13:492-496.

305. Milligan WL, Powell DA, Harley C, Furchtgott E. A comparison of physical health and psychosocial variables as predictors of reaction time and serial learning performance in elderly men. J Gerontol 1984;39:704-710.

306. Berger BG, Friedmann E, Eaton M. Comparison of jogging, the relaxation response, and group interaction for stress reduction. J Sport Exerc Psychol 1988;10:434-447.

307. Berger BG, Owen DR. Mood alteration with swimming - swimmers really do "feel better." Psychosom Med 1983;45:425-433.

308. Berger BG, Owen DR. Anxiety reduction with swimming: Relationships between exercise and state, trait, and somatic anxiety. Int J Sport Psychol 1987;18:286-302.

309. Berger BG, Owen DR. Mood alteration with yoga and swimming: Aerobic exercise may not be necessary.

Percept Mot Skills 1992;75:1331-1343.

310. Krause N, Goldenhar L, Liang J, Jay G, Maeda D. Stress and exercise among the Japanese elderly. Soc Sci Med 1993;36:1429-1441.

311. Harma MI, Ilmarinen J, Knauth P. Physical training intervention in female shift workers: II. The effects of intervention on the circadian rhythms of alertness, short-term memory, and body temperature. Ergonomics 1988;31:51-63.

312. Raglin JS. Exercise and mental health. Beneficial and detrimental effects. Sports Med 1990;9:323-329.

313. Head A, Kendall MJ, Ferner R, Eagles C. Acute effects of b blockade and exercise on mood and anxiety. Br J Sports Med 1996;30:238-242.

314. Gannon L, Luchetta T, Pardie L, Rhodes K. Perimenstrual symptoms: Relationships with chronic stress and selected lifestyle variables. J Behav Med 1989;12:149-159.

315. Keye WR. Medical treatment of premenstrual syndrome. Can J Psychiatr 1985;30:483-487.

316. Schwartz B, Cumming DC, Riordan E, Selye M, Yen SS, Rebar RW. Exercise-associated amenorrhea: A distinct entity? Am J Obstet Gynecol 1981;141:662-670.

317. Palinkas LA, Barrett-Connor E. Estrogen use and depressive symptoms in postmenopausal women. Obstet Gynecol 1992;80:30-36.

318. Palinkas LA, Wingard DL, Barrett-Connor E. Depressive

symptoms in overweight and obese older adults: A test of the "jolly fat" hypothesis. J Psychosom Res 1996;40:59-66.

319. Cooper-Patrick L, Ford DE, Mead LA, Chang PP, Klag MJ. Exercise and depression in mid-life: A prospective study. Am J Public Health 1997;87:670-673.

320. Craft LL, Landers DM. The effect of exercise on clinical depression: A meta-analysis [abstract]. Med Sci Sports Exerc 1998;30(Suppl 5):S117.

321. Cramer SR, Neiman DC, Lee JW. The effects of moderate exercise training on psychological well-being and mood state in women. J Psychosom Res 1991;35:437-449.

322. King AC, Taylor CB, Haskell WL, De Busk RF. Influence of regular aerobic exercise on psychological health: A randomized, controlled trial of healthy, middle-aged adults. Health Psychol 1989;8:305-324.

323. Larson E, Wang M, et al. Exercise Is Associated with Reduced Risk for Incident Dementia among Persons 65 Years of Age and Older. Annals of Internal Medicine, 17 January 2006 | Volume 144 Issue 2 | Pages 73-81.

324. Laurin D, Verreault R, Lindsay J, MacPherson K, Rockwood K. Physical activity and risk of cognitive impair- ment and dementia in elderly persons. Arch Neurol. 2001 Mar;58(3):498-504.

325. Li G, Shen YC, Chen CH, Zhau YW, Li SR, Lu M. A three-year follow-up study of age-related dementia

in an urban area of Beijing. Acta Psychiatr Scand 1991;83:99-104.

326. Mayeux R, Ottman R, Tang MX, Noboa-Bauza L, Marder K, Gurland B, Stern Y. Genetic susceptibility and head injury as risk factors for Alzheimer's disease among community-dwelling elderly persons and their first-degree relatives. Ann Neurol 1993;33:494-501.

327. Smith C, Rose GM. Evidence for a paradoxical sleep window for place learning in the Morris water maze. Physiol Behav 1996;59:93-97.

328. Smith C, Rose GM. Posttraining paradoxical sleep in rats is increased after spatial learning in the Morris water maze. Behav Neurosci 1997;111:1197-1204.

329. Fishbein W. Disruptive effects of rapid eye movement sleep deprivation on long-term memory. Physiol Behav 1971;6:279-282.

330. Pearlman CA, Greenberg R. Posttrial REM sleep: A critical period for consolidation of shuttlebox avoidance. Animal Learn Behav 1973;1:49-51.

331. Smith CT, Conway JM, Rose GM. Brief paradoxical sleep deprivation impairs reference, but not working, memory in the radial arm maze task. Neurobiol Learn Memory 1998;69:211-217.

332. Bourtchouladze R, Abel T, Berman N, Gordon R, Lapidus K, Kandel ER. Different training procedures for contextual memory in mice can recruit either one or two critical periods for memory consolidation that require protein synthesis and PKA. Learn Memory

1998;5:365-374.

333. Abel T, Nguyen PV, Barad M, Deuel TA, Kandel ER, Bourtchouladze R. Genetic demonstration of a role for PKA in the late phase of LTP and in hippocampus-based long-term memory. Cell 1997;88:615-626.

334. Smith CT, Tenn C, Annett R. Some biochemical and behavioural aspects of the paradoxical sleep window. Can J Psychol 1991;45:115-124.

335. Marrosu F, Portas C, Mascia MS, Casu MA, Fa M, Giagheddu M, Imperato A, Gessa GL. Microdialysis measurement of cortical and hippocampal acetylcholine release during sleep-wake cycle in freely moving cats. Brain Res 1995;671:329-332.

336. Graves L, Pack A, Abel T. Sleep and memory: A molecular perspective. Trends Neurosci 2001;24:237- 243.

337. Auerbach JM, Segal M. A novel cholinergic induction of long-term potentiation in rat hippocampus. J Neurophysiol 1994;72:2034-2040.

338. Matsuyama S, Matsumoto A, Enomoto T, Nishizaki T. Activation of nicotinic acetylcholine receptors induces long-term potentiation in vivo in the intact mouse dentate gyrus. Eur J Neurosci 2000;12:3741-3747.

339. King AC, Oman RF, Brassington GS, Bliwise DL, Haskell WL. Moderate-intensity exercise and self-rated quality of sleep in older adults. A randomized

controlled trial. JAMA. 1997 Jan 1;277(1):32-7.

340. Li F, Fisher KJ, Harmer P, Irbe D, Tearse RG, Weimer C. Tai chi and self-rated quality of sleep and daytime sleepiness in older adults: a randomized controlled trial. J Am Geriatr Soc. 2004 Jun;52(6):892-900.

341. King AC, Baumann K, O'Sullivan P, Wilcox S, Castro C. Effects of moderate-intensity exercise on physiological, behavioral, and emotional responses to family caregiving: a randomized controlled trial. J Gerontol A Biol Sci Med Sci. 2002 Jan;57(1):M26-36.

342. Singh NA, Clements KM, Fiatarone MA. A randomized controlled trial of the effect of exercise on sleep. Sleep. 1997 Feb;20(2):95-101.

343. Tworoger SS, Yasui Y, Vitiello MV, et al. Effects of a yearlong moderate-intensity exercise and a stretching intervention on sleep quality in postmenopausal women. Sleep. 2003 Nov 1;26(7):830-6.

344. Lira FS, et al. Exercise training improves sleep pattern and metabolic profile in elderly people in a time-dependent manner. Lipids Health Dis. 2011 July 6;10:1-6.

345. Flausino NH, et al. Physical exercise performed before bedtime improves the sleep pattern of healthy young good sleepers. Psychopharmacology. 2012 Feb;49(2):186-92.

346. Monteleone P, Beinat L, Tanzillo C, Maj M, Kemali D. Effects of phosphatidylserine on the neuroendocrine response to physical stress in humans. Neuroendocri-

nology 1990;52:243-248.

347. Benton D, Donohoe RT, Sillance B, Nabb S. The influence of phosphatidylserine supplementation on mood and heart rate when faced with an acute stressor. Nutr Neurosci 2001;4:169-178.

348. Hellhammer J, Fries E, Buss C, Engert V, Tuch A, Rutenberg D, Hellhammer D. Effects of soy lecithin phosphatidic acid and phosphatidylserine complex (PAS) on the endocrine and psychological responses to mental stress. Stress 2004;7:119-126.

349. Monteleone P, Maj M, Beinat L, Natale M, Kemali D. Blunting by chronic phosphatidylserine administration of the stress-induced activation of the hypothalamo-pituitary-adrenal axis in healthy men. Eur J Clin Pharmacol 1992;41:385-388.

350. Fahey TD, Pearl MS. The hormonal and perceptive effects of phosphatidylserine administration during two weeks of resistive exercise-induced overtraining. Biol Sport 1998;15:135-144.

351. Jäger R, Purpura M, Geiss KR, Weiß M, Baumeister J, Amatulli F, Schröder L, Herwegen H. The effect of phosphatidylserine on golf performance. J Int Soc Sports Nutr 2007;4:23.

352. Starks MA, Starks SL, Kingsley M, Purpura M, Jäger R. The effects of phosphatidylserine on endocrine response to moderate intensity exercise. J Int Soc Sports Nutr 2008;5:11 (doi: 10.1186/1550-2783-5-

11).

353. Singh A, Petrides JS, Gold PW, Chrousos GP, Deuster PA. Differential hypothalamic-pituitary-adrenal axis reactivity to psychological and physical stress. J Clin Endocrinol Metab 1999;84:1944-1948.

354. Goto S, Kogure K, Abe K, Kimata Y, Kitahama K, Yamashita E, Terada H. Efficient radical trapping at the surface and inside the phospholipid membrane is responsible for highly potent antiperoxidative activity of the carotenoid astaxanthin. Biochim Biophys Acta 2001;1512:251-258.

355. Beutner S, Bloedorn B, Frixel S, Hernandez Blanco I, Hoffmann T, Martin H-D, Mayer B, Noack P, Ruck C, Schmidt M, Schulke I, Sell S, Ernst H, Haremza S, Seybold G, Sies H, Stahl W, Walsh R. Quantitative assessment of antioxidant properties of natural colorants and phytochemicals: Carotenoids, flavonoids, phenols and indigoids. The role of ?-carotene in antioxidant functions. J Sci Food Agric 2001;81:559-568.

356. Shimidzu N, Goto M, Miki W. Carotenoids as singlet oxygen quenchers in marine organisms. Fish Sci 1996;62:134-137.

357. Nishida Y, Yamashita E, Miki W. Quenching activities of common hydrophilic and lipophilic antioxidants against singlet oxygen using chemiluminescence detection system. Carotenoid Sci 2007;11:16-20.

358. Di Mascio P, Devasagayam TP, Kaiser S, Sies H. Carot-

enoids, tocopherols and thiols as biological singlet molecular oxygen quenchers. Biochem Soc Trans 1990;18:1054-1056.

359. Bagchi D. Oxygen free radical scavenging abilities of vitamins C, E, ?-carotene, pycnogenol, grape seed proanthocyanidin extract and astaxanthins in vitro. Unpublished data, 2001.

360. Kobayashi M, Kakizono T, Nishio N, Nagai S, Kurimura Y, Tsuji Y. Antioxidant role of astaxanthin in the green alga Haematococcus pluvialis. Appl Microbiol Biotechnol 1997;48:351-356.

361. Bell JG, McEvoy J, Tocher DR, Sargent JR. Depletion of ?-tocopherol and astaxanthin in Atlantic salmon (Salmo salar) affects autoxidative defense and fatty acid metabolism. J Nutr 2000;130:1800-1808.

362. Palozza P, Krinsky NI. Astaxanthin and canthaxanthin are potent antioxidants in a membrane model. Arch Biochem Biophys 1992;297:291-295.

363. McNulty H, Jacob RF, Mason RP. Biologic activity of carotenoids related to distinct membrane physico-chemical interactions. Am J Cardiol 2008;101:20D-29D.

364. McNulty HP, Byun J, Lockwood SF, Jacob RF, Mason RP. Differential effects of carotenoids on lipid peroxidation due to membrane interactions: X-ray diffraction analysis. Biochim Biophys Acta 2007;1768:167-174.

365. Mason RP, Walter MF, McNulty HP, Lockwood SF, Byun

J, Day CA, Jacob RF. Rofecoxib increases susceptibility of human LDL and membrane lipids to oxidative damage: A mechanism of cardiotoxicity. J Cardiovasc Pharmacol 2006;47(Suppl. 1):S7-S14.

366. Woodall AA, Britton G, Jackson MJ. Carotenoids and protection of phospholipids in solution or in liposomes against oxidation by peroxyl radicals: Relationship between carotenoid structure and protective ability. Biochim Biophys Acta 1997;1336:575-586.

367. Lim BP, Nagao A, Terao J, Tanaka K, Suzuki T, Takama K. Antioxidant activity of xanthophylls on peroxyl radical-mediated phospholipid peroxidation. Biochim Biophys Acta 1992;1126:178-184.

368. Nakagawa K, Kang SD, Park DK, Handelman GJ, Miyazawa T. Inhibition of ?- carotene and astaxanthin of NADPH-dependent microsomal phospholipid peroxidation. J Nutr Sci Vitaminol 1997;43:345-355.

369. Iwamoto T, Hosoda K, Hirano R, Kurata H, Matsumoto A, Miki W, Kamiyama M, Itakura H, Yamamoto S, Kondo K. Inhibition of low-density lipoprotein oxidation by astaxanthin. J Atheroscler Thromb 2000;7:216-222.

370. Guerin M, Huntley ME, Olaizola M. Haematococcus astaxanthin: Applications for human health and nutrition. Trends Biotechnol 2003;21:210-216.

371. Hayakawa T, Kulkarni A, Terada Y, Maoka T, Etoh H. Reaction of astaxanthin with peroxynitrite. Biosci

Biotechnol Biochem 2008;72:2716-2722.

372. Etoh H, Suhara M, Tokuyama S, Kato H, Nakahigashi R, Maejima Y, Ishikura M, Terada Y, Maoka T. Auto-oxidation products of astaxanthin. J Oleo Sci 2012;61:17-21.

373. Guerra BA, Otton R. Impact of the carotenoid astaxanthin on phagocytic capacity and ROS/RNS production of human neutrophils treated with free fatty acids and high glucose. Int Immunopharmacol 2011;11:2220-2226.

374. Hama S, Uenishi S, Yamada A, Ohgita T, Tsuchiya H, Yamashita E, Kogure K. Scavenging of hydroxyl radicals in aqueous solution by astaxanthin encapsulated in liposomes. Biol Pharm Bull 2012;35:2238-2242.

375. Maoka T, Tokuda H, Suzuki N, Kato H, Etoh H. Antioxidative, anti-tumor- promoting, and anti-carcinogensis activities of nitroastaxanthin and nitrolutein, the reaction products of astaxanthin and lutein with peroxynitrite. Mar Drugs 2012;10:1391-1399.

376. Rodrigues E, Mariutti LR, Mercadante AZ. Scavenging capacity of marine carotenoids against reactive oxygen and nitrogen species in a membrane-mimicking system. Mar Drugs 2012;10:1784-1798.

377. Khan SK, Malinski T, Mason RP, Kubant R, Jacob RF, Fujioka K, Denstaedt SJ, King TJ, Jackson HL, Hieber AD, Lockwood SF, Goodin TH, Pashkow FJ, Bodary PF. Novel astaxanthin prodrug (CDX-085) attenuates thrombosis in a mouse

model. Thromb Res 2010;Aug 20 (doi:10.1016/j. thromres.2010.07.003).

378. Kurashige M, Okimasu E, Inoue M, Utsumi K. Inhibition of oxidative injury of biological membranes by astaxanthin. Physiol Chem Phys Med NMR. 1990;22:27- 38.

379. Nishigaki I, Rajendran P, Venugopal R, Ekambaram G, Sakthisekaran D, Nishigaki

Y. Cytoprotective role of astaxanthin against glycated protein/iron chelate-induced toxicity in human umbilical vein endothelial cells. Phytother Res 2010;24:54-59.

380. Comhaire FH, El Garem Y, Mahmoud A, Eertmans F, Schoonjans F. Combined conventional/antioxidant "Astaxanthin" treatment for male infertility: A double blind, randomized trial. Asian J Androl 2005;7:257-262.

381. Kudo Y, Nakjima R, Matsumoto N, Tsukahara H. Effects of astaxanthin on brain damages due to ischemia. Carotenoid Sci 2002;5:25.

382. Kim JH, Choi W, Lee JH, Jeon SJ, Choi YH, Kim BW, Chang HI, Nam SW.

Astaxanthin inhibits H2O2-mediated apoptotic cell death in mouse neural progenitor cells via modulation of P38 and MEK signaling pathways. J Microbiol Biotechnol 2009;19:1355-1363.

383. Asami S, Yang Z-B, Yamashita E, Otoze H. Anti-stress

composition. United States patent US 6265450. US Patent and Trademark Office, Alexandria, VA, 2001, 15 pages.

384. Kim JH, Kim YS, Song GG, Park JJ, Chang HI. Protective effect of astaxanthin on naproxen-induced gastric antral ulceration in rats. Eur J Pharmacol 2005;514:53- 59.

385. Lee DH, Kim CS, Lee YJ. Astaxanthin protects against MPTP/MPP+-induced mitochondrial dysfunction and ROS production in vivo and in vitro. Food Chem Toxicol 2011;49:271-280.

386. Dong LY, Jin J, Lu G, Kang XL. Astaxanthin attenuates the apoptosis of retinal ganglion cells in db/db mice by inhibition of oxidative stress. Mar Drugs 2013;11:960-974.

387. Augusti PR, Quatrin A, Somacal S, Conterato GM, Sobieski R, Ruviaro AR, Maurer LH, Duarte MM, Roehrs M, Emanuelli T. Astaxanthin prevents changes in the activities of thioredoxin reductase and paraoxonase in hypercholesterolemic rabbits. J Clin Biochem Nutr 2012;51:42-49.

388. O'Connor I, O'Brien N. Modulation of UVA light-induced oxidative stress by ?- carotene, lutein and astaxanthin in cultured fibroblasts. J Dermatol Sci 1998;16:226-230.

389. Lyons NM, O'Brien NM. Modulatory effects of an algal extract containing astaxanthin on UVA-irradiated

cells in culture. J Dermatol Sci 2002;30:73-84.

390. Choi HD, Kim JH, Chang MJ, Kyu-Youn Y, Shin WG. Effects of astaxanthin on oxidative stress in overweight and obese adults. Phytother Res 2011a;25:1813- 1818.

391. Choi HD, Youn YK, Shin WG. Positive effects of astaxanthin on lipid profiles and oxidative stress in overweight subjects. Plant Foods Hum Nutr 2011b;66:363-369.

392. Jacobs AT, Marnett LJ. Systems analysis of protein modification and cellular responses induced by electrophile stress. Acc Chem Res 2010;43:673-683.

393. Romero FJ, Bosch-Morell F, Romero MJ, Jareño EJ, Romero B, Marín N, Romá J. Lipid peroxidation products and antioxidants in human disease . Environ Health Perspect 1998;106 (Suppl. 5):1229-1234.

394. Kim YK, Chyun J-H. The effects of astaxanthin supplements on lipid peroxidation and antioxidant status in postmenopausal women. Nutr Sci 2004;7:41-46.

395. Iwabayashi M, Fujioka N, Nomoto K, Miyazaki R, Takahashi H, Hibino S, Takahashi Y, Nishikawa K, Nishida M, Yonei Y. Efficacy and safety of eight-week treatment with astaxanthin in individuals screened for increased oxidative stress burden. J Anti-Aging Med 2009;6:15-21.

396. Park JS, Chyun JH, Kim YK, Line LL, Chew BP. Astaxanthin decreased oxidative stress and inflammation

and enhanced immune response in humans. Nutr Metab 2010;7:18 (http://www.nutritionandmetabolism.com/content/7/1/18).

397. Mertens-Talcott SU, Jilma-Stohlawetz P, Rios J, Hingorani L, Derendorf H. Absorption, metabolism, and antioxidant effects of pomegranate (Punica granatum l.) polyphenols after ingestion of a standardized extract in healthy human volunteers. J Agric Food Chem 2006;54:8956-8961.

398. Tzulker R, Glazer I, Bar-Ilan I, Holland D, Aviram M, Amir R. Antioxidant activity, polyphenol content, and related compounds in different fruit juices and homogenates prepared from 29 different pomegranate accessions. J Agric Food Chem 2007;55:9559-9570.

399. Gil MI, Tomás-Barberán FA, Hess-Pierce B, Holcroft DM, Kader AA. Antioxidant activity of pomegranate juice and its relationship with phenolic composition and processing. J Agric Food Chem 2000;48:4581-4589.

400. Colombo E, Sangiovanni E, Dell'agli M. A review on the anti-inflammatory activity of pomegranate in the gastrointestinal tract. Evid Based Complement Alternat Med 2013;2013:247145 (doi: 10.1155/2013/247145).

401. Elfalleh W, Hannachi H, Tlili N, Yahia Y, Nasri N, Ferchichi A. Total phenolic contents and antioxidant activities of pomegranate peel, seed, leaf and flower. J

Med Plants Res 2012;6:4724-4730.

402. Seeram NP, Aronson WJ, Zhang Y, Henning SM, Moro A, Lee RP, Sartippour M, Harris DM, Rettig M, Suchard MA, Pantuck AJ, Belldegrun A, Heber D. Pomegranate ellagitannin-derived metabolites inhibit prostate cancer growth and localize to the mouse prostate gland. J Agric Food Chem 2007 19;55:7732-7737.

403. Seeram NP, Henning SM, Zhang Y, Suchard M, Li Z, Heber D. Pomegranate juice ellagitannin metabolites are present in human plasma and some persist in urine for up to 48 hours. J Nutr 2006;136:2481-2485.

404. Adams LS, Zhang Y, Seeram NP, Heber D, Chen S. Pomegranate ellagitannin- derived compounds exhibit antiproliferative and antiaromatase activity in breast cancer cells in vitro. Cancer Prev Res 2010;3:108-113.

405. Yoshida T, Amakura Y, Yoshimura M. Structural features and biological properties of ellagitannins in some plant families of the order myrtales. Int J Mol Sci 2010;11:79-106.

406. Del Rio D, Rodriguez-Mateos A, Spencer JP, Tognolini M, Borges G, Crozier A. Dietary (poly)phenolics in human health: structures, bioavailability, and evidence of protective effects against chronic diseases. Antioxid Redox Signal 2013;18:1818- 1892.

407. Seeram NP, Zhang Y, McKeever R, Henning SM, Lee

RP, Suchard MA, Li Z, Chen S, Thames G, Zerlin A, Nguyen M, Wang D, Dreher M, Heber D. Pomegranate juice and extracts provide similar levels of plasma and urinary ellagitannin metabolites in human subjects. J Med Food 2008;11:390-394.

408. Aviram M, Rosenblat M, Gaitini D, Nitecki S, Hoffman A, Dornfeld L, Volkova N, Presser D, Attias J, Liker H, Hayek T. Pomegranate juice consumption for 3 years by patients with carotid artery stenosis reduces common carotid intima-media thickness, blood pressure and LDL oxidation. Clin Nutr 2004;23:423-433.

409. Gözlekçi S, Saraço?lu O, Onursal E, Ozgen M. Total phenolic distribution of juice, peel, and seed extracts of four pomegranate cultivars. Pharmacogn Mag 2011;7:161-164.

410. González-Sarrías A, Giménez-Bastida JA, García-Conesa MT, Gómez-Sánchez MB, García-Talavera NV, Gil-Izquierdo A, Sánchez-Alvarez C, Fontana-Compiano LO, Morga-Egea JP, Pastor-Quirante FA, Martínez-Díaz F, Tomás-Barberán FA, Espín JC. Occurrence of urolithins, gut microbiota ellagic acid metabolites and proliferation markers expression response in the human prostate gland upon consumption of walnuts and pomegranate juice. Mol Nutr Food Res 2010;54:311- 322.

411. Pantuck AJ, Leppert JT, Zomorodian N, Aronson W, Hong J, Barnard RJ, Seeram N, Liker H, Wang H, Elashoff R, Heber D, Aviram M, Ignarro L, Belldeg-

run A. Phase II study of pomegranate juice for men with rising prostate-specific antigen following surgery or radiation for prostate cancer. Clin Cancer Res 2006;12:4018- 4026.

412. Kulkarni AP, Mahal HS, Kapoor S, Aradhya SM. In vitro studies on the binding, antioxidant, and cytotoxic actions of punicalagin. J Agric Food Chem 2007;55:1491-1500.

413. Anonymous. Pomegranate 40p. P.I. Thomas & Co., Inc., Morristown NJ, undated, unpaged.

414. Shukla M, Gupta K, Rasheed Z, Khan KA, Haqqi TM. Bioavailable constituents/metabolites of pomegranate (Punica granatum L) preferentially inhibit COX2 activity ex vivo and IL-1?-induced PGE2 production in human chondrocytes in vitro. J Inflamm 2008;5:9.

415. Lansky EP, Newman RA. Punica granatum (pomegranate) and its potential for prevention and treatment of inflammation and cancer. J Ethnopharmacol 2007;109:177-206.

416. Elfalleh W, Tlili N, Nasri N, Yahia Y, Hannachi H, Chaira N, Ying M, Ferchichi A. Antioxidant capacities of phenolic compounds and tocopherols from Tunisian pomegranate (Punica granatum) fruits. J Food Sci 2011;76:C707-C713.

417. Seeram NP, Aviram M, Zhang Y, Henning SM, Feng L, Dreher M, Heber D. Comparison of antioxidant potency of commonly consumed polyphenol-rich beverages in the United States. J Agric Food Chem

2008;56:1415-1422.

418. Carlsen MH, Halvorsen BL, Holte K, Bøhn SK, Drag-
      land S, Sampson L, Willey C, Senoo H, Umezono Y,
      Sanada C, Barikmo I, Berhe N, Willett WC, Phillips
      KM, Jacobs DR Jr, Blomhoff R. The total antioxidant
      content of more than 3100 foods, beverages, spices,
      herbs and supplements used worldwide. Nutr J
      2010;9:3 (doi: 10.1186/1475-2891-9-3).

419. Carlsen MH, Halvorsen BL, Holte K, Bøhn SK, Drag-
      land S, Sampson L, Willey C, Senoo H, Umezono
      Y, Sanada C, Barikmo I, Berhe N, Willett WC,
      Phillips KM, Jacobs DR Jr, Blomhoff R. The total
      antioxidant content of more than 3100 foods, bever-
      ages, spices, herbs and supplements used worldwide.
      Additional File 1. Nutr J 2010;9:3, 138 pages (doi:
      10.1186/1475-2891-9-3).

420. Rosenblat M, Volkova N, Attias J, Mahamid R, Aviram
      M. Consumption of polyphenolic-rich beverages
      (mostly pomegranate and black currant juices) by
      healthy subjects for a short term increased serum
      antioxidant status, and the serum's ability to attenuate
      macrophage cholesterol accumulation. Food Funct
      2010a;1:99- 109.

421. Draganov DI, Teiber JF, Speelman A, Osawa Y, Suna-
      hara R, La Du BN. Human paraoxonases (PON1,
      PON2, and PON3) are lactonases with overlap-
      ping and distinct substrate specificities. J Lipid Res

2005;46:1239-1247.

422. Aviram M, Rosenblat M. Pomegranate protection against cardiovascular diseases. Evid Based Complement Alternat Med 2012;2012:382763 (doi: 10.1155/2012/382763).

423. Aqil F, Munagala R, Vadhanam MV, Kausar H, Jeyabalan J, Schultz DJ, Gupta RC. Anti-proliferative activity and protection against oxidative DNA damage by punicalagin isolated from pomegranate husk. Food Res Int 2012;49:345-353.

424. Fuhrman B, Partoush A, Volkova N, Aviram M. Ox-LDL induces monocyte-to- macrophage differentiation in vivo: Possible role for the macrophage colony stimulating factor receptor (M-CSF-R). Atherosclerosis 2008;196:598-607.

425. Rosenblat M, Volkova N, Coleman R, Aviram M. Pomegranate byproduct administration to apolipoprotein E-deficient mice attenuates atherosclerosis development as a result of decreased macrophage oxidative stress and reduced cellular uptake of oxidized low-density lipoprotein. J Agric Food Chem 2006;54:1928-1935.

426. Rosenblat M, Volkova N, Aviram M. Pomegranate juice (PJ) consumption antioxidative properties on mouse macrophages, but not PJ beneficial effects on macrophage cholesterol and triglyceride metabolism, are mediated via PJ-induced stimulation of macrophage

PON2. Atherosclerosis 2010b;212:86-92.

427. Shiner M, Fuhrman B, Aviram M. Macrophage paraoxonase 2 (PON2) expression is up-regulated by pomegranate juice phenolic anti-oxidants via PPAR?and AP-1 pathway activation. Atherosclerosis 2007;195:313-321.

428. Ng CJ, Wadleigh DJ, Gangopadhyay A, Hama S, Grijalva VR, Navab M, Fogelman AM, Reddy ST. Paraoxonase-2 is a ubiquitously expressed protein with antioxidant properties and is capable of preventing cell-mediated oxidative modification of low density lipoprotein. J Biol Chem 2001;276:44444-44449.

429. Ng CJ, Wadleigh DJ, Gangopadhyay A, Hama S, Grijalva VR, Navab M, Fogelman AM, Reddy ST. Paraoxonase-2 is a ubiquitously expressed protein with antioxidant properties and is capable of preventing cell-mediated oxidative modification of low density lipoprotein. J Biol Chem 2001;276:44444-44449.

430. de Nigris F, Williams-Ignarro S, Sica V, Lerman LO, D'Armiento FP, Byrns RE, Casamassimi A, Carpentiero D, Schiano C, Sumi D, Fiorito C, Ignarro LJ, Napoli C. Effects of a pomegranate fruit extract rich in punicalagin on oxidation-sensitive genes and eNOS activity at sites of perturbed shear stress and atherogenesis. Cardiovasc Res 2007;73:414-423.

431. de Nigris F, Williams-Ignarro S, Lerman LO, Crimi E, Botti C, Mansueto G, D'Armiento FP, De Rosa G, Sica V, Ignarro LJ, Napoli C. Beneficial effects of

pomegranate juice on oxidation-sensitive genes and endothelial nitric oxide synthase activity at sites of perturbed shear stress. Proc Natl Acad Sci U S A 2005;102:4896-4901.

432. Sestili P, Martinelli C, Ricci D, Fraternale D, Bucchini A, Giamperi L, Curcio R, Piccoli G, Stocchi V. Cytoprotective effect of preparations from various parts of Punica granatum L. fruits in oxidatively injured mammalian cells in comparison with their antioxidant capacity in cell free systems. Pharmacol Res 2007;56:18-26.

433. Bialonska D, Kasimsetty SG, Khan SI, Ferreira D. Urolithins, intestinal microbial metabolites of Pomegranate ellagitannins, exhibit potent antioxidant activity in a cell-based assay. J Agric Food Chem 2009;57:10181-10186.

434. Bhattacharya T, Nicholls SJ, Topol EJ, Zhang R, Yang X, Schmitt D, Fu X, Shao M, Brennan DM, Ellis SG, Brennan ML, Allayee H, Lusis AJ, Hazen SL. Relationship of paraoxonase 1 (PON1) gene polymorphisms and functional activity with systemic oxidative stress and cardiovascular risk. JAMA 2008; 299: 1265- 1276.

435. Aviram M, Dornfeld L, Rosenblat M, Volkova N, Kaplan M, Coleman R, Hayek T, Presser D, Fuhrman B. Pomegranate juice consumption reduces oxidative stress, atherogenic modifications to LDL, and platelet aggregation: Studies in humans and in atherosclerotic apolipoprotein E-deficient mice. Am J Clin Nutr

2000;71:1062- 1076.

436. Gaidukov L, Tawfik DS. The development of human sera tests for HDL-bound serum PON1 and its lipolactonase activity. J Lipid Res 2007;48:1637-1646.

437. Watson AD, Berliner JA, Hama SY, La Du BN, Faull KF, Fogelman AM, Navab

M. Protective effect of high density lipoprotein associated paraoxonase. Inhibition of the biological activity of minimally oxidized low density lipoprotein. J Clin Invest 1995;96:2882-2891.

438. Aviram M, Billecke S, Sorenson R, Bisgaier C, Newton R, Rosenblat M, Erogul J, Hsu C, Dunlop C, La Du B. Paraoxonase active site required for protection against LDL oxidation involves its free sulfhydryl group and is different from that required for its arylesterase/paraoxonase activities: Selective action of human paraoxonase allozymes Q and R. Arterioscler Thromb Vasc Biol 1998;18:1617-1624.

439. Mackness MI, Arrol S, Durrington PN. Paraoxonase prevents accumulation of lipoperoxides in low-density lipoprotein. FEBS Lett 1991;286:152-154.

440. Rosenblat M, Gaidukov L, Khersonsky O, Vaya J, Oren R, Tawfik DS, Aviram M. The catalytic histidine dyad of high density lipoprotein-associated serum paraoxonase-1 (PON1) is essential for PON1-mediated inhibition of low density lipoprotein oxidation and stimulation of macrophage cholesterol efflux. J Biol

Chem 2006;281:7657-7665.

441. Costa LG, Giordano G, Furlong CE. Pharmacological and dietary modulators of paraoxonase 1 (PON1) activity and expression: The hunt goes on. Biochem Pharmacol 2011;81:337-344.

442. Litvinov D, Mahini H, Garelnabi M. Antioxidant and anti-inflammatory role of paraoxonase 1: Implication in arteriosclerosis diseases. N Am J Med Sci 2012;4:523-532.

443. Rock W, Rosenblat M, Miller-Lotan R, Levy AP, Elias M, Aviram M. Consumption of wonderful variety pomegranate juice and extract by diabetic patients increases paraoxonase 1 association with high-density lipoprotein and stimulates its catalytic activities. J Agric Food Chem 2008;56:8704-8713.

444. Slater TF, Sawyer BC. The stimulatory effects of carbon tetrachloride and other halogenoalkanes on peroxidative reactions in rat liver fractions in vitro. General features of the systems used. Biochem J 1971;123:805-814.

445. Tomita I, Sano M, Serizawa S, Ohta K, Katou M. Fluctuation of lipid peroxides and related enzyme activities at time of stroke in stroke-prone spontaneously hypertensive rats. Stroke 1979;10:323-326.

446. Parsaeyan N, Mozaffari-Khosravi H, Mozayan MR. Effect of pomegranate juice on paraoxonase enzyme activity in patients with type 2 diabetes. J Diabetes Metab Disord 2012;11:11 (doi: 10.1186/2251-6581-

11-11).

447. Balbir-Gurman A, Fuhrman B, Braun-Moscovici Y, Markovits D, Aviram M. Consumption of pomegranate decreases serum oxidative stress and reduces disease activity in patients with active rheumatoid arthritis: A pilot study. Isr Med Assoc J 2011;13:474-479.

448. Rosenblat M, Hayek T, Aviram M. Anti-oxidative effects of pomegranate juice (PJ) consumption by diabetic patients on serum and on macrophages. Atherosclerosis 2006;187:363-371.

449. Davidson MH, Maki KC, Dicklin MR, Feinstein SB, Witchger M, Bell M, McGuire DK, Provost JC, Liker H, Aviram M. Effects of consumption of pomegranate juice on carotid intima-media thickness in men and women at moderate risk for coronary heart disease. Am J Cardiol 2009;104:936-942.

450. Shema-Didi L, Sela S, Ore L, Shapiro G, Geron R, Moshe G, Kristal B. One year of pomegranate juice intake decreases oxidative stress, inflammation, and incidence of infections in hemodialysis patients: A randomized placebo-controlled trial. Free Radic Biol Med 2012;53:297-304.

451. Sumner MD, Elliott-Eller M, Weidner G, Daubenmier JJ, Chew MH, Marlin R, Raisin CJ, Ornish D. Effects of pomegranate juice consumption on myocardial perfusion in patients with coronary heart disease. Am J Cardiol 2005;96:810-814.

452. Taddei S, Galetta F, Virdis A, Ghiadoni L, Salvetti G,

Franzoni F, Giusti C, Salvetti A. Physical activity prevents age-related impairment in nitric oxide availability in elderly athletes. Circulation 2000;101:2896-2901.

453. Taddei S, Virdis A, Ghiadoni L, Salvetti G, Bernini G, Magagna A, Salvetti A. Age-related reduction of NO availability and oxidative stress in humans. Hypertension 2001;38:274-279.

454. Mauras N, O'Brien KO, Klein KO, Hayes V. Estrogen suppression in males: Metabolic effects. J Clin Endocrinol Metab 2000;85:2370-2377.

455. Burnett-Bowie SA, McKay EA, Lee H, Leder BZ. Effects of aromatase inhibition on bone mineral density and bone turnover in older men with low testosterone levels. J Clin Endocrinol Metab 2009;94:4785-4792.

456. Balunas MJ, Kinghorn AD. Natural compounds with aromatase inhibitory activity: An update. Planta Med 2010;76:1087-1093.

457. Wang L, Ho J, Glackin C, Martins-Green M. Specific pomegranate juice components as potential inhibitors of prostate cancer metastasis. Transl Oncol 2012;5:344-355.

458. Adhami VM, Khan N, Mukhtar H. Cancer chemoprevention by pomegranate: Laboratory and clinical evidence. Nutr Cancer 2009;61:811-815.

459. Bell C, Hawthorne S. Ellagic acid, pomegranate and prostate cancer -- a mini review. J Pharm Pharmacol

2008;60:139-144.

460. Malik A, Mukhtar H. Prostate cancer prevention through pomegranate fruit. Cell Cycle 2006;5:371-373.

461. Malik A, Afaq F, Sarfaraz S, Adhami VM, Syed DN, Mukhtar H. Pomegranate fruit juice for chemoprevention and chemotherapy of prostate cancer. Proc Natl Acad Sci U S A 2005;102:14813-14818.

462. Koyama S, Cobb LJ, Mehta HH, Seeram NP, Heber D, Pantuck AJ, Cohen P. Pomegranate extract induces apoptosis in human prostate cancer cells by modulation of the IGF-IGFBP axis. Growth Horm IGF Res 2010;20:55-62.

463. Albrecht M, Jiang W, Kumi-Diaka J, Lansky EP, Gommersall LM, Patel A, Mansel RE, Neeman I, Geldof AA, Campbell MJ. Pomegranate extracts potently suppress proliferation, xenograft growth, and invasion of human prostate cancer cells. J Med Food 2004;7:274-283.

464. Hong MY, Seeram NP, Heber D. Pomegranate polyphenols down-regulate expression of androgen-synthesizing genes in human prostate cancer cells overexpressing the androgen receptor. J Nutr Biochem 2008;19:848-855.

465. Rettig MB, Heber D, An J, Seeram NP, Rao JY, Liu H, Klatte T, Belldegrun A, Moro A, Henning SM, Mo D, Aronson WJ, Pantuck A. Pomegranate extract inhibits androgen-independent prostate cancer growth through a nuclear factor-?B- dependent mechanism.

Mol Cancer Ther 2008;7:2662-2671.

466. Sartippour MR, Seeram NP, Rao JY, Moro A, Harris DM, Henning SM, Firouzi A, Rettig MB, Aronson WJ, Pantuck AJ, Heber D. Ellagitannin-rich pomegranate extract inhibits angiogenesis in prostate cancer in vitro and in vivo. Int J Oncol 2008;32:475-480.

467. Adhami VM, Siddiqui IA, Syed DN, Lall RK, Mukhtar H. Oral infusion of pomegranate fruit extract inhibits prostate carcinogenesis in the TRAMP model. Carcinogenesis 2012;33:644-651.

468. Paller CJ, Ye X, Wozniak PJ, Gillespie BK, Sieber PR, Greengold RH, Stockton BR, Hertzman BL, Efros MD, Roper RP, Liker HR, Carducci MA. A randomized phase II study of pomegranate extract for men with rising PSA following initial therapy for localized prostate cancer. Prostate Cancer Prostatic Dis 2013;16:50- 55.

469. Wallace TC. Anthocyanins in cardiovascular disease. Adv Nutr 2011;2:1-7.

470. de Pascual-Teresa S, Moreno DA, García-Viguera C. Flavanols and anthocyanins in cardiovascular health: A review of current evidence. Int J Mol Sci 2010;11:1679-1703.

471. Mazza GJ. Anthocyanins and heart health. Ann Ist Super Sanita 2007;43:369-374.

472. Galvano F, La Fauci L, Vitaglione P, Fogliano V, Vanella L, Felgines C. Bioavailability, antioxidant and biolog-

ical properties of the natural free-radical scavengers cyanidin and related glycosides. Ann Ist Super Sanita 2007;43:382-393.

473. Ding M, Feng R, Wang SY, Bowman L, Lu Y, Qian Y, Castranova V, Jiang BH, Shi X. Cyanidin-3-glucoside, a natural product derived from blackberry, exhibits chemopreventive and chemotherapeutic activity. J Biol Chem 2006;281:17359- 17368.

474. Fukumoto LR, Mazza G. Assessing antioxidant and prooxidant activities of phenolic compounds. J Agric Food Chem 2000;48:3597-3604.

475. Kolodziej H, Kayser O, Kiderlen AF, Ito H, Hatano T, Yoshida T, Foo LY. Proanthocyanidins and related compounds: Antileishmanial activity and modulatory effects on nitric oxide and tumor necrosis factor-?-release in the murine macrophage-like cell line RAW 264.7. Biol Pharm Bull 2001;24:1016-1021.

476. Noda Y, Kaneyuki T, Mori A, Packer L. Antioxidant activities of pomegranate fruit extract and its anthocyanidins: Delphinidin, cyanidin, and pelargonidin. J Agric Food Chem 2002;50:166-171.

477. Ichiyanagi T, Hatano Y, Matsugo S, Konishi T. Kinetic comparisons of anthocyanin reactivities towards 2,2'-azobis(2-amidinopropane) (AAPH) radicals, hydrogen peroxide and tert-buthylhydroperoxide by capillary zone electrophoresis. Chem Pharm Bull 2004;52:434-438.

478. Kano M, Takayanagi T, Harada K, Makino K, Ishikawa

F. Antioxidative activity of anthocyanins from purple sweet potato, Ipomoera batatas cultivar Ayamurasaki. Biosci Biotechnol Biochem 2005;69:979-988.

479. Cao G, Prior RL. Comparison of different analytical methods for assessing total antioxidant capacity of human serum. Clin Chem 1998;44:1309-1315.

480. Wang CC, Chu CY, Chu KO, Choy KW, Khaw KS, Rogers MS, Pang CP. Trolox- equivalent antioxidant capacity assay versus oxygen radical absorbance capacity assay in plasma. Clin Chem 2004;50:952-954.

481. Ohnishi R, Ito H, Kasajima N, Kaneda M, Kariyama R, Kumon H, Hatano T, Yoshida T. Urinary excretion of anthocyanins in humans after cranberry juice ingestion. Biosci Biotechnol Biochem 2006;70:1681-1687.

482. Cao G, Prior RL. Anthocyanins are detected in human plasma after oral administration of an elderberry extract. Clin Chem 1999;45:574-576.

483. Cao G, Muccitelli HU, Sánchez-Moreno C, Prior RL. Anthocyanins are absorbed in glycated forms in elderly women: A pharmacokinetic study. Am J Clin Nutr 2001;73:920-926.

484. Del Rio D, Borges G, Crozier A. Berry flavonoids and phenolics: Bioavailability and evidence of protective effects. Br J Nutr 2010;104(Suppl. 3):S67-S90.

485. Kay CD, Mazza G, Holub BJ, Wang J. Anthocyanin metabolites in human urine and serum. Br J Nutr.

2004;91:933-942.

486. Mazza G, Kay CD, Cottrell T, Holub BJ. Absorption of anthocyanins from blueberries and serum antioxidant status in human subjects. J Agric Food Chem 2002;50:7731-7737.

487. Mazza G, Kay CD. Bioactivity, absorption, and metabolism of anthocyanins. In: Lattanzio V, Daayf F (eds.). Recent Advances in Polyphenols Research. Vol. I. Blackwell Publishing Ltd., Oxford, UK 2008, pp. 228-262.

488. Talavéra S, Felgines C, Texier O, Besson C, Manach C, Lamaison JL, Rémésy C. Anthocyanins are efficiently absorbed from the small intestine in rats. J Nutr 2004;134:2275-2279.

489. Spormann TM, Albert FW, Rath T, Dietrich H, Will F, Stockis JP, Eisenbrand G, Janzowski C. Anthocyanin/polyphenolic-rich fruit juice reduces oxidative cell damage in an intervention study with patients on hemodialysis. Cancer Epidemiol Biomarkers Prev 2008;17:3372-3380.

490. Hafeez BB, Siddiqui IA, Asim M, Malik A, Afaq F, Adhami VM, Saleem M, Din M, Mukhtar H. A dietary anthocyanidin delphinidin induces apoptosis of human prostate cancer PC3 cells in vitro and in vivo: Involvement of nuclear factor-?B signaling. Cancer Res 2008;68:8564-8572.

491. Hafeez BB, Asim M, Siddiqui IA, Adhami VM, Murtaza I, Mukhtar H. Delphinidin, a dietary anthocy-

anidin in pigmented fruits and vegetables: A new weapon to blunt prostate cancer growth. Cell Cycle 2008;7:3320-3326.

492. Nandakumar V, Singh T, Katiyar SK. Multi-targeted prevention and therapy of cancer by proanthocyanidins. Cancer Lett 2008;269:378-387.

493. Calderón AI, Wright BJ, Hurst WJ, van Breemen RB. Screening antioxidants using LC-MS: Case study with cocoa. J Agric Food Chem 2009;57:5693-5699.

494. Lee YA, Cho EJ, Tanaka T, Yokozawa T. Inhibitory activities of proanthocyanidins from persimmon against oxidative stress and digestive enzymes related to diabetes. J Nutr Sci Vitaminol 2007;53:287-292.

495. Kimura Y, Ito H, Kawaji M, Ikami T, Hatano T. Characterization and antioxidative properties of oligomeric proanthocyanidin from prunes, dried fruit of Prunus domestica L. Biosci Biotechnol Biochem 2008;72:1615-1618.

496. Osakabe N, Yasuda A, Natsume M, Takizawa T, Terao J, Kondo K. Catechins and their oligomers linked by C4 ? C8 bonds are major cacao polyphenols and protect low-density lipoprotein from oxidation in vitro. Exp Biol Med 2002;227:51-56.

497. Hashimoto F, Ono M, Masuoka C, Ito Y, Sakata Y, Shimizu K, Nonaka G, Nishioka I, Nohara T. Evaluation of the anti-oxidative effect (in vitro) of tea polyphenols. Biosci Biotechnol Biochem 2003;67:396-

401.

498. Rein D, Lotito S, Holt RR, Keen CL, Schmitz HH, Fraga CG. Epicatechin in human plasma: In vivo determination and effect of chocolate consumption on plasma oxidation status. J Nutr 2000;130(Suppl.):2109S-2114S.

499. Wang JF, Schramm DD, Holt RR, Ensunsa JL, Fraga CG, Schmitz HH, Keen CL. A dose-response effect from chocolate consumption on plasma epicatechin and oxidative damage. J Nutr 2000;130(Suppl.):2115S-2119S.

500. Wan Y, Vinson JA, Etherton TD, Proch J, Lazarus SA, Kris-Etherton PM. Effects of cocoa powder and dark chocolate on LDL oxidative susceptibility and prostaglandin concentrations in humans. Am J Clin Nutr.2001;74:596-602.

501. Sano A, Uchida R, Saito M, Shioya N, Komori Y, Tho Y, Hashizume N. Beneficial effects of grape seed extract on malondialdehyde-modified LDL. J Nutr Sci Vitaminol 2007;53:174-182.

502. De Marzo AM, Platz EA, Sutcliffe S, Xu J, Grönberg H, Drake CG, Nakai Y, Isaacs WB, Nelson WG. Inflammation in prostate carcinogenesis. Nat Rev Cancer 2007;7:256-269.

503. Billis A. Prostatic atrophy. Clinicopathological signifi-

cance. Int Braz J Urol 2010;36:401-409.

504. De Marzo AM, Marchi VL, Epstein JI, Nelson WG. Proliferative inflammatory atrophy of the prostate: Implications for prostatic carcinogenesis. Am J Pathol 1999;155:1985-1992.

505. Pathak SK, Sharma RA, Steward WP, Mellon JK, Griffiths TRL, Gescher AJ. Oxidative stress and cyclooxygenase activity in prostate carcinogenesis: Targets for chemopreventive strategies. Eur J Cancer 2005;41:61-70.

506. Majumder PK, Yeh JJ, George DJ, Febbo PG, Kum J, Xue Q, Bikoff R, Ma H-F, Kantoff PW, Golub TR, Loda M, Sellers WR. Prostate intraepithelial neoplasia induced by prostate restricted Akt activation: The MPAKT model. Proc Natl Acad Sci USA 2003;100:7841-7846.

507. Greenberg NM, Demayo F, Finegold MJ, Medina D, Tilley WD, Aspinall JO, Cunha GR, Donjacour AA, Matusik RJ, Rosen JM. Prostate cancer in a transgenic mouse. Proc Natl Acad Sci USA 1995;92:3439-3443.

508. Christov KT, Moon RC, Lantvit DD, Boone CW, Steele VE, Lubet RA, Kelloff GJ, Pezzuto JM. 9-cis-Retinoic aid but not 4-(hydroxyphenyl)retinamide inhibits prostate intraepithelial neoplasia in Noble rats. Cancer Res 2002;62:5178-5182.

509. Huang JP, Powell WC, Khodavirdi AC, Wu J, Makita T,

Cardiff RD, Cohen MB, Sucov HM, Roy-Burman P. Prostatic intraepithelial neoplasia in mice with conditional disruption of the Retinoid X Receptor ? allele in the prostate epithelium. Cancer Res 2002;62:4812-4819.

510. Montironi R, Mazzucchelli R, Marshall JR, Bartels PH. Prostate cancer prevention: Review of target populations, pathological biomarkers, and chemopreventive agents. J Clin Pathol 1999;52;793-803.

511. Montironi R, Mazzucchelli R, Algaba F, Lopez-Beltran A. Morphological identification of the patterns of prostatic intraepithelial neoplasia and their importance. J Clin Pathol 2000;53;655-665.

512. Park J-H, Walls JE, Galvez JJ, Kim M, Abate-Shen C, Shen MM, Cardiff RD. Prostatic intraepithelial neoplasia in genetically engineered mice. Am J Pathol 2002, 161:727–735.

513. Reiter RE, Gu Z, Watabe T, Thomas G, Szigeti K, Davis E, Wahl M, Nisitani S, Yamashiro J, Le Beau MM, Loda M, Witte ON. Prostate stem cell antigen: A cell surface marker overexpressed in prostate cancer. Proc Natl Acad Sci USA 1998;95:1735-1740.

514. Marnett LJ. Oxyradicals and DNA damage. Carcinogenesis 2000;21:361-370.

515. Beckman KB, Ames BN. Oxidative decay of DNA. J Biol Chem 1997;272:19633-19636.

516. Lenton KJ, Therriault H, Fulop T, Payette H, Wagner RJ. Glutathione and ascorbate are negatively correlated

with oxidative DNA damage in human lymphocytes. Carcinogenesis 1999;20:607-613.

517. Martinet W, Knaapen MWM, De Meyer GRY, Herman AG, Kock MM. Oxidative DNA damage and repair in experimental atherosclerosis are reversed by dietary lipid lowering. Circ Res 2001;88:733-739.

518. Guzder SN, Torres-Ramos C, Johnson RE, Haracska L, Prakash L, Prakash S. Requirement of yeast Rad1– Rad10 nuclease for the removal of 3'-blocked termini from DNA strand breaks induced by reactive oxygen species. Genes Devel 2004;18:2283-2291.

519. Luo Y, Han Z, Chin SM, Linn S. Three chemically distinct types of oxidants formed by iron-mediated Fenton reactions in the presence of DNA. Proc Natl Acad Sci USA 1994;91:12438-12442.

520. Keyer K, Imlay JA. Superoxide accelerates DNA damage by elevating free- iron levels. Proc Natl Acad Sci USA 1996;93:13635-13640.

521. Henle ES, Linn S. Formation, prevention, and repair of DNA damage by iron/hydrogen peroxide. J Biol Chem 1997;272:19095-19098.

522. Beckman JS, Beckman TW, Chen J, Marshall PA, Freeman BA. Apparent hydroxyl radical production by peroxynitrite: Implications for endothelial injury from nitric oxide and superoxide. Proc Natl Acad Sci U S A 1990;87:1620-1624.

523. Jaruga P, Dizdaroglu M. Repair of products of oxidative DNA base damage in human cells. Nucleic Acids Res

1996;24:1389-1394.

524. Johnson TM, Yut Z-X, Ferrans VJ, Lowenstein RA, Finkel T. Reactive oxygen species are downstream mediators of p53-dependent apoptosis. Proc Natl Acad Sci U S A 1996;93:11848-11852.

525. Cheng KC, Cahill DS, Kasai H, Nishimura S, Loeb LA. 8-Hydroxyguanine, an abundant form of oxidative DNA damage, causes G?T and A?C substitutions. J Biol Chem 1992;267:166-172.

526. Moriya M. Single-stranded shuttle phagemid for muta-genesis studies in mammalian cells: 8-oxoguanine in DNA induces targeted G•C?T•A transversions in simian kidney cells. Proc Natl Acad Sci U S A 1993;90:1122-1126.

527. Kreutzer DA, Essigmann JM. Oxidized, deaminated cytosines are a source of C?T transitions in vivo. Proc Natl Acad Sci U S A 1998;95:3578-3582.

528. Sharma RA, Farmer PB. Biological relevance of adduct detection to the chemoprevention of cancer. Clin Cancer Res 2004;10:4901-4912.

529. Malins DC, Polissar NL, Ostrander GK, Vinson MA. Single 8-oxo-guanine and 8- oxo-adenine lesions induce marked changes in the backbone structure of a 25-base DNA strand. Proc Natl Acad Sci U S A 2000;97:12442-12445.

530. Gedik CM, Boyle SP, Wood SG, Vaughan NJ, Collins AR. Oxidative stress in humans: Validation of biomarkers of DNA damage. Carcinogenesis

2002;23:1441-1446.

531. Fink SP, Reddy GR, Marnett LJ. Mutagenicity in Escherichia coli of the major DNA adduct derived from the endogenous mutagen malondialdehyde. Proc Natl Acad Sci USA 1997;94:8652-8657.

532. Henle ES, Luo Y, Gassmann W, Linn S. Oxidative damage to DNA constituents by iron-mediated Fenton reactions. The deoxyguanosine family. J Biol Chem 1996;271:21177-21186.

533. Luo Y, Henle ES, Linn S. Oxidative damage to DNA constituents by iron-mediated Fenton reactions. The deoxycytidine family. J Biol Chem 1996;271:21167-21176.

534. Cheng KC, Preston BD, Cahill DS, Dosanjh MK, Singer B, Loeb LA. The vinyl chloride DNA derivative N2,3-ethenoguanine produces G?A transitions in Escherichia coli. Proc Natl Acad Sci U S A 1991;88:9974-9978.

535. Moriya M, Zhang W, Johnson F, Grollman AP. Mutagenic potency of exocyclic DNA adducts: Marked differences between Escherichia coli and simian kidney cells. Proc Natl Acad Sci U S A 1994;91:11899-11903.

536. Nath RG, Chung FL. Detection of exocyclic 1,N2-propanodeoxyguanosine adducts as common DNA lesions in rodents and humans. Proc Natl Acad Sci U S A 1994;91:7491-7495.

537. Hagen TM, Huang S, Curnutte J, Fowler P, Martinez V,

Wehr CM, Ames BN, Chisari FV. Extensive oxidative DNA damage in hepatocytes of transgenic mice with chronic active hepatitis destined to develop hepatocellular carcinoma. Proc Natl Acad Sci U S A 1994;91:12808-12812.

538. Farinati F, Cardin R, Degan P, Rugge M, Mario FD, Bonvicini P, Naccarato R. Oxidative DNA damage accumulation in gastric carcinogenesis. Gut 1998;42:351- 356.

539. Adelman R, Saul RL, Ames BN. Oxidative damage to DNA: Relation to species metabolic rate and life span. Proc Natl Acad Sci USA 1988;85:2706-2708.

540. Malins DC, Polissar NL, Gunselman SJ. Models of DNA structure achieve almost perfect discrimination between normal prostate, benign prostatic hyperplasia (BPH), and adenocarcinoma and have a high potential for predicting BPH and prostate cancer. Proc Natl Acad Sci USA 1997;94:259-264.

541. Malins DC, Johnson PM, Wheeler TM, Barker EA, Polissar NL, Vinson MA. Age- related radical-induced DNA damage is linked to prostate cancer. Cancer Res 2001;61:6025-6028.

542. Rushmore TH, Pickett CB. Glutathione S-transferases: Structure, regulation, and therapeutic implications. J Biol Chem 1993;268:11475-11478.

543. Cooke MS, Evans MD, Dizdaroglu M, Lunec J. Oxidative DNA damage: Mechanisms, mutation, and

disease. FASEB J 2003;17:1195-1214.

544. Marks LS, Mazer NA, Mostaghel E, Hess DL, Dorey FJ, Epstein JI, Veltri RW, Makarov DV, Partin AW, Bostwick DG, Macairan ML, Nelson PS. Effect of testosterone replacement therapy on prostate tissue in men with late-onset hypogonadism: A randomized controlled trial. JAMA 2006;296:2351-2361.

545. Cherrier MM, Matsumoto AM, Amory JK, Johnson M, Craft S, Peskind ER, Raskind MA. Characterization of verbal and spatial memory changes from moderate to supraphysiological increases in serum testosterone in healthy older men. Psychoneuroendocrinology 2007;32:72-79.

546. Kenny AM, Kleppinger A, Annis K, Rathier M, Browner B, Judge JO, McGee D. Effects of transdermal testosterone on bone and muscle in older men with low bioavailable testosterone levels, low bone mass, and physical frailty. J Am Geriatr Soc 2010;58:1134-1143.

547. Basaria S, Coviello AD, Travison TG, Storer TW, Farwell WR, Jette AM, Eder R, Tennstedt S, Ulloor J, Zhang A, Choong K, Lakshman KM, Mazer NA, Miciek R, Krasnoff J, Elmi A, Knapp PE, Brooks B, Appleman E, Aggarwal S, Bhasin G, Hede-Brierley L, Bhatia A, Collins L, LeBrasseur N, Fiore LD, Bhasin S. Adverse events associated with testosterone administration. N Engl J Med 2010;363:109- 122.

548. Sih R, Morley JE, Kaiser FE, Perry HM 3rd, Patrick P,

Ross C. Testosterone replacement in older hypogonadal men: A 12-month randomized controlled trial. J Clin Endocrinol Metab 1997;82:1661-1667.

549. Bhasin S, Woodhouse L, Casaburi R, Singh AB, Bhasin D, Berman N, Chen X, Yarasheski KE, Magliano L, Dzekov C, Dzekov J, Bross R, Phillips J, Sinha-Hikim I, Shen R, Storer TW. Testosterone dose-response relationships in healthy young men. Am J Physiol Endocrinol Metab 2001;281:E1172-E1181.

550. Wang C, Swerdloff RS, Iranmanesh A, Dobs A, Snyder PJ, Cunningham G, Matsumoto AM, Weber T, Berman N; Testosterone Gel Study Group. Transdermal testosterone gel improves sexual function, mood, muscle strength, and body composition parameters in hypogonadal men. J Clin Endocrinol Metab 2000;85:2839-2853.

551. Jeong SM, Ham BK, Park MG, Oh MM, Yoon DK, Kim JJ, Moon du G. Effect of testosterone replacement treatment in testosterone deficiency syndrome patients with metabolic syndrome. Korean J Urol 2011;52:566-571.

552. Hero M, Ankarberg-Lindgren C, Taskinen MR, Dunkel L. Blockade of oestrogen biosynthesis in peripubertal boys: Effects on lipid metabolism, insulin sensitivity, and body composition. Eur J Endocrinol 2006;155:453-460.

553. Lapauw B, T'Sjoen G, Mahmoud A, Kaufman JM, Ruige JB. Short-term aromatase inhibition: Effects on

glucose metabolism and serum leptin levels in young and elderly men. Eur J Endocrinol 2009;160:397-402.

554. Kawakami J, Morales A. Clinical significance of suboptimal hormonal levels in men with prostate cancer treated with LHRH agonists. Can Urol Assoc J 2013;7:E226-E230.

555. Hsing AW, Comstock GW. Serological precursors of cancer: Serum hormones and risk of subsequent prostate cancer. Cancer Epidemiol Biomarkers Prev 1993;2:27- 32.

556. Chen C, Weiss NS, Stanczyk FZ, Lewis SK, DiTommaso D, Etzioni R, Barnett MJ, Goodman GE. Endogenous sex hormones and prostate cancer risk: A case-control study nested within the Carotene and Retinol Efficacy Trial. Cancer Epidemiol Biomarkers Prev 2003;12:1410-1416.

557. de Jong FH, Oishi K, Hayes RB, Bogdanowicz JF, Raatgever JW, van der Maas PJ, Yoshida O, Schroeder FH. Peripheral hormone levels in controls and patients with prostatic cancer or benign prostatic hyperplasia: Results from the Dutch-Japanese case-control study. Cancer Res 1991;51:3445-3450.

558. Pechersky AV, Mazurov VI, Semiglazov VF, Karpischenko AI, Mikhailichenko VV, Udintsev AV. Androgen administration in middle-aged and ageing men: Effects of oral testosterone undecanoate on dihydrotestosterone, oestradiol and prostate volume. Int J Androl

2002;25:119-125.

559. Ramasamy R, Fisher ES, Schlegel PN. Testosterone replacement and prostate cancer. Indian J Urol 2012;28:123-128.

560. Wirén S, Stattin P. Androgens and prostate cancer risk. Best Pract Res Clin Endocrinol Metab 2008;22:601-613.

561. Bain J. The many faces of testosterone. Clin Interv Aging. 2007;2:567-576.

562. Bosland MC, Mahmoud AM. Hormones and prostate carcinogenesis: Androgens and estrogens. J Carcinog 2011;10:116-125.

563. Morgentaler A . Testosterone and prostate cancer: An historical perspective on a modern myth. Eur Urol 2006;50:935-939.

564. Eaton NE, Reeves GK, Appleby PN, Key TJ. Endogenous sex hormones and prostate cancer: A quantitative review of prospective studies. Br J Cancer 1999;80:930-934.

565. Mulligan T, Frick MF, Zuraw QC, Stemhagen A, McWhirter C. Prevalence of hypogonadism in males aged at least 45 years: The HIM study. Int J Clin Pract 2006;60:762-769.

566. Fernández-Balsells MM, Murad MH, Lane M, Lampropulos JF, Albuquerque F, Mullan RJ, Agrwal N, Elamin MB, Gallegos-Orozco JF, Wang AT, Erwin PJ, Bhasin S, Montori VM. Clinical review 1:

Adverse effects of testosterone therapy in adult men: A systematic review and meta-analysis. J Clin Endocrinol Metab 2010;95:2560-2575.

567. Buvat J, Maggi M, Gooren L, Guay AT, Kaufman J, Morgentaler A, Schulman C, Tan HM, Torres LO, Yassin A, Zitzmann M. Endocrine aspects of male sexual dysfunctions. J Sex Med 2010;7:1627-1656.

568. Buvat J, Maggi M, Guay A, Torres LO. Testosterone deficiency in men: Systematic review and standard operating procedures for diagnosis and treatment. J Sex Med 2013;10:245-284.

569. Wang C, Nieschlag E, Swerdloff R, Behre HM, Hellstrom WJ, Gooren LJ, Kaufman JM, Legros JJ, Lunenfeld B, Morales A, Morley JE, Schulman C, Thompson IM, Weidner W, Wu FC. ISA, ISSAM, EAU, EAA and ASA recommendations: Investigation, treatment and monitoring of late-onset hypogonadism in males. Int J Impot Res 2009;21:1-8.